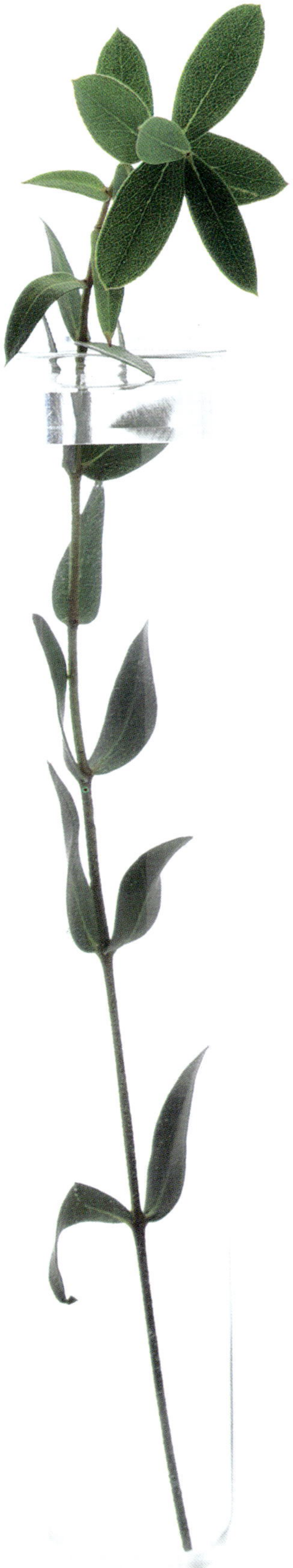

# AROMATHERAPY MASSAGE FOR YOU

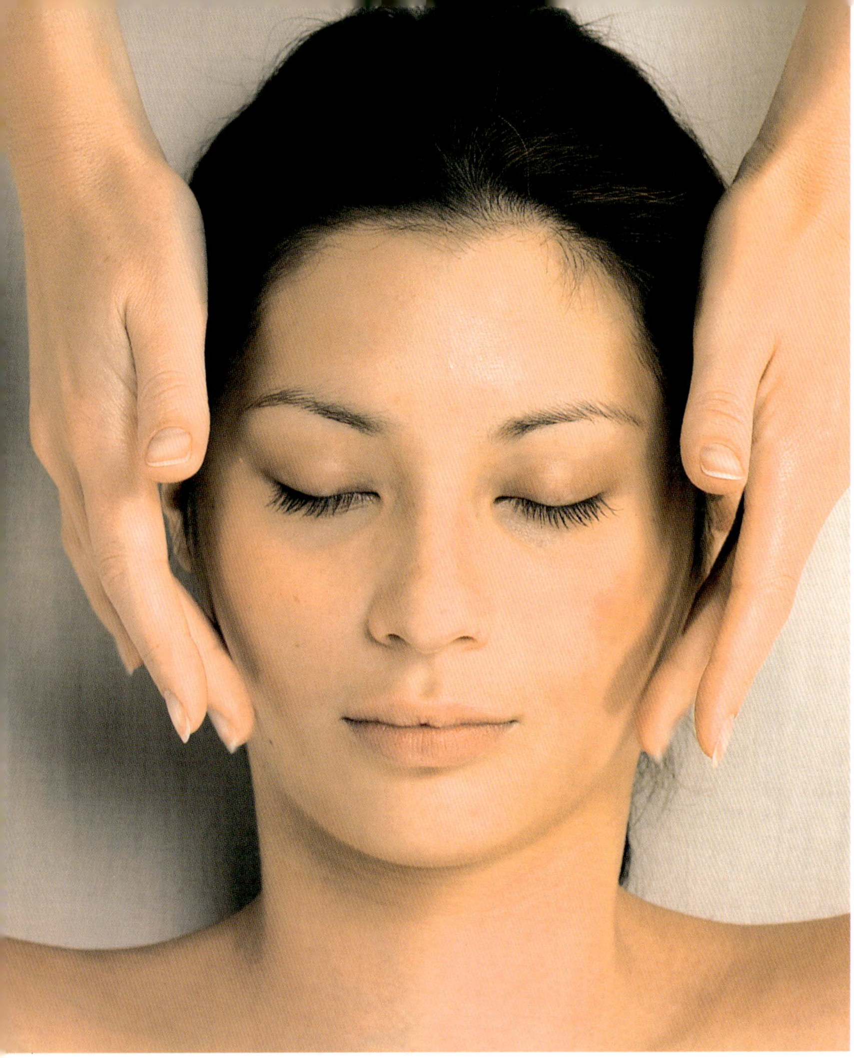
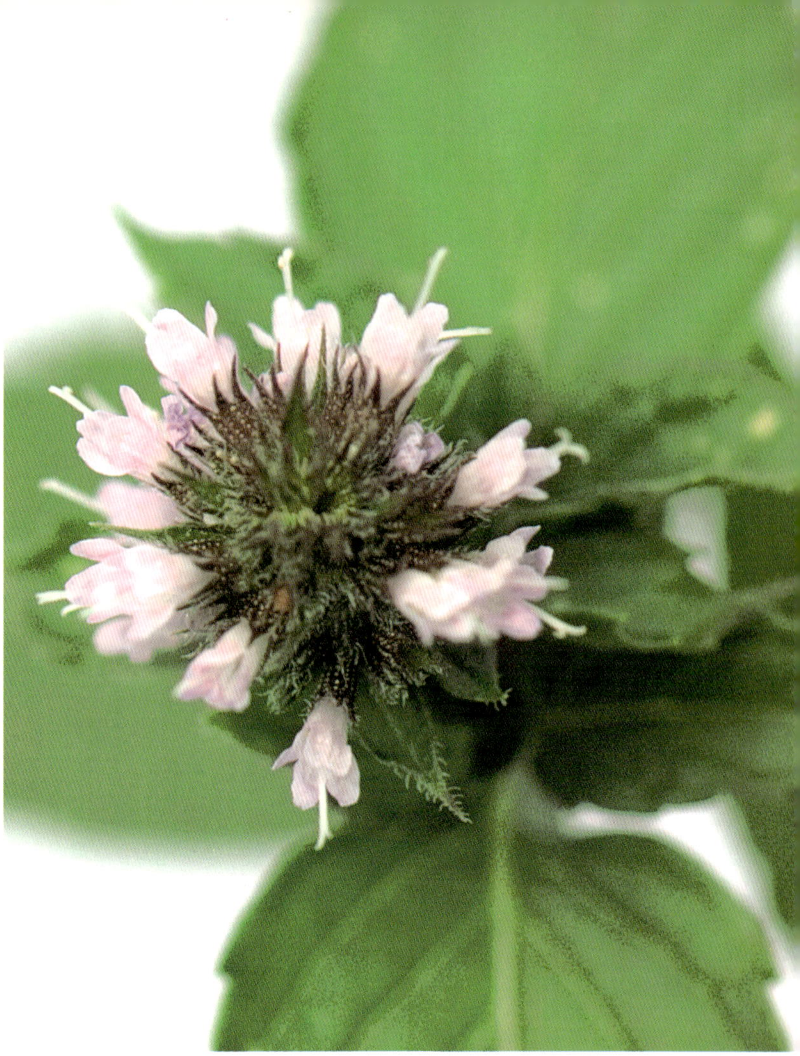
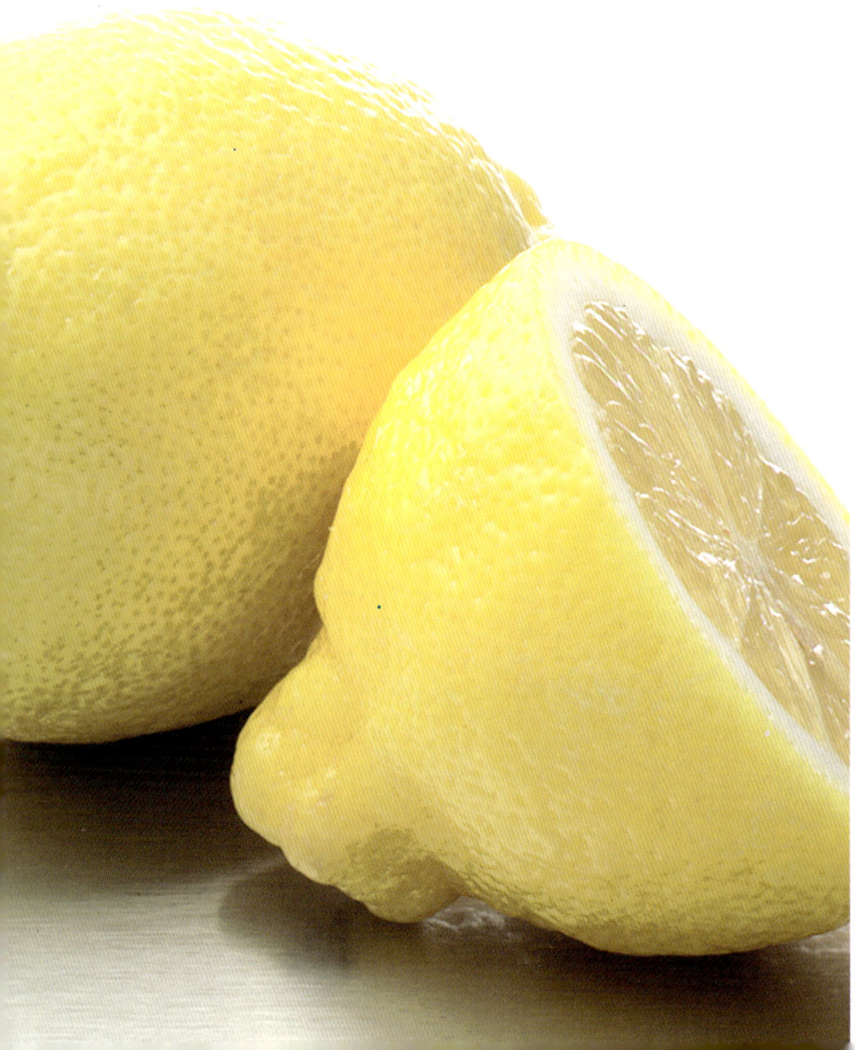
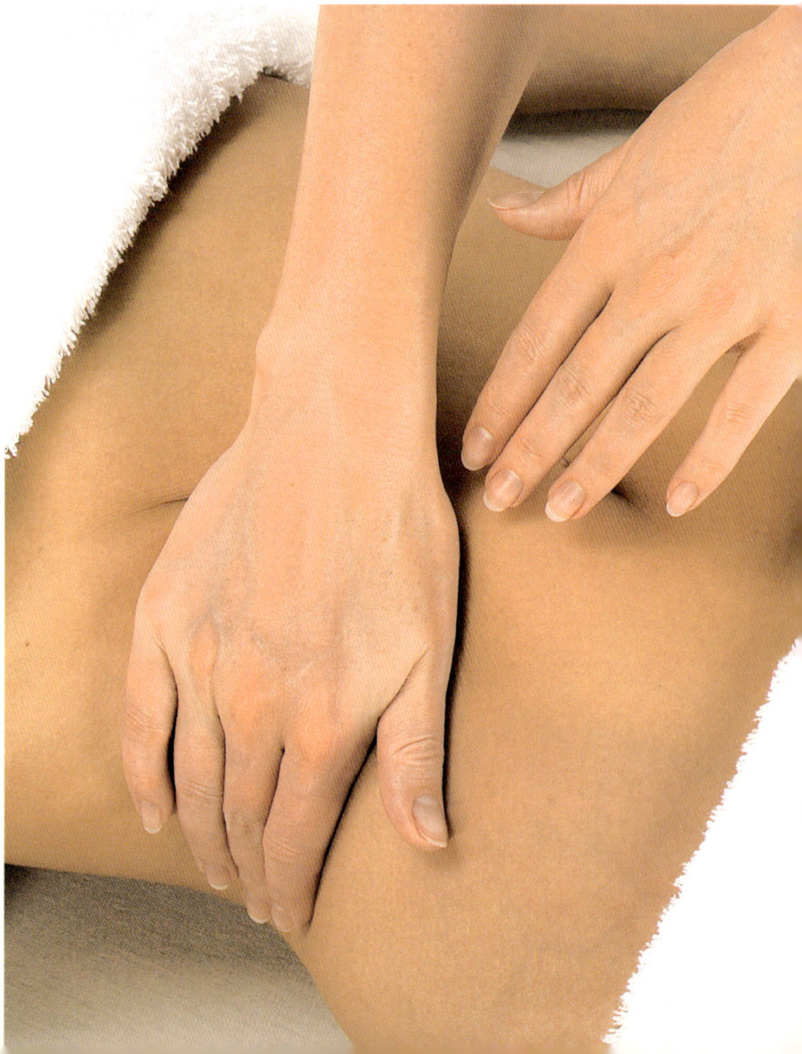

JENNIE HARDING

# AROMATHERAPY MASSAGE FOR YOU

THE PRACTICAL STEP-BY-STEP GUIDE TO AROMATHERAPY MASSAGE AT HOME

DUNCAN BAIRD PUBLISHERS

LONDON

This book is dedicated to my mother and father, Sonja and John Harding, with love.

**Aromatherapy Massage for You**
Jennie Harding

First published in the United Kingdom and Ireland in 2005 by
Duncan Baird Publishers Ltd
Sixth Floor
Castle House
75–76 Wells Street
London W1T 3QH

Conceived, created and designed by
Duncan Baird Publishers



Managing Editor: Julia Charles
Editors: Rebecca Miles with Ingrid Court-Jones
Managing Designer: Manisha Patel
Designer: Rachel Cross
Picture Researcher: Louise Glasson
Commissioned photography: Matthew Ward (people) and William Lingwood (plants)

British Library Cataloguing-in-Publication Data:
A CIP record for this book is available from the British Library

10 9 8 7 6 5 4 3 2 1

ISBN-10: 1-84483-144-2 ISBN-13: 9-781844-831449

Typeset in Helvetica Neue
Colour reproduction by Scanhouse, Malaysia
Printed in Singapore by Imago

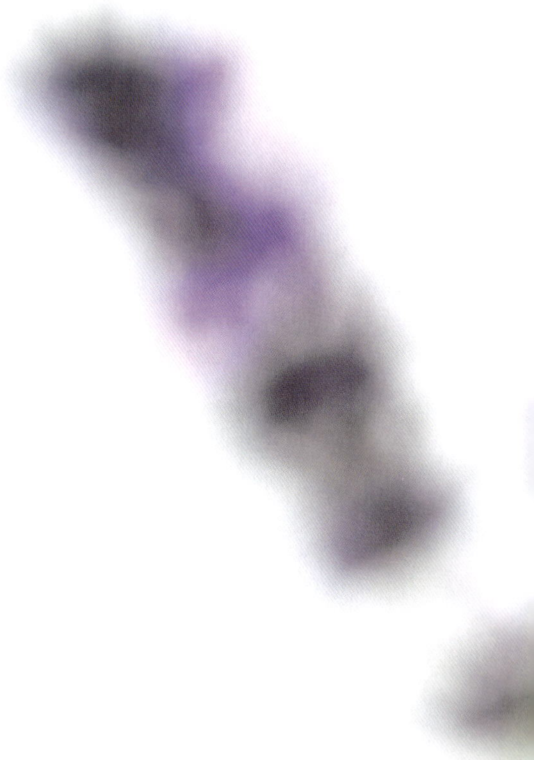

Note on abbreviations:
BCE (Before the Common Era) is the equivalent of BC.
CE (Common Era) is the equivalent of AD.

*"Look in the perfumes of flowers and of Nature for peace of mind and joy of life."*

Wang Wei (8th century CE)

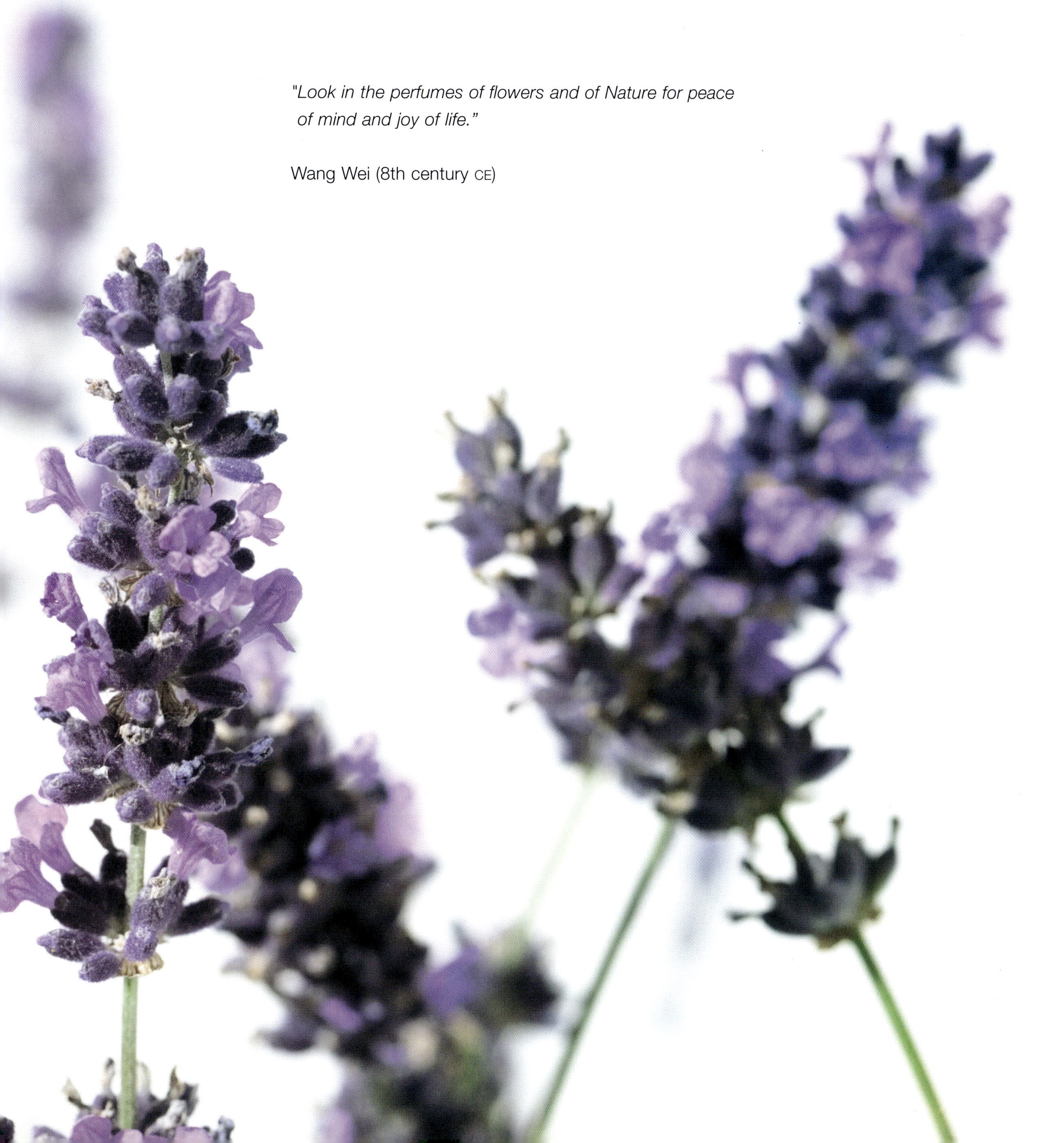

# contents

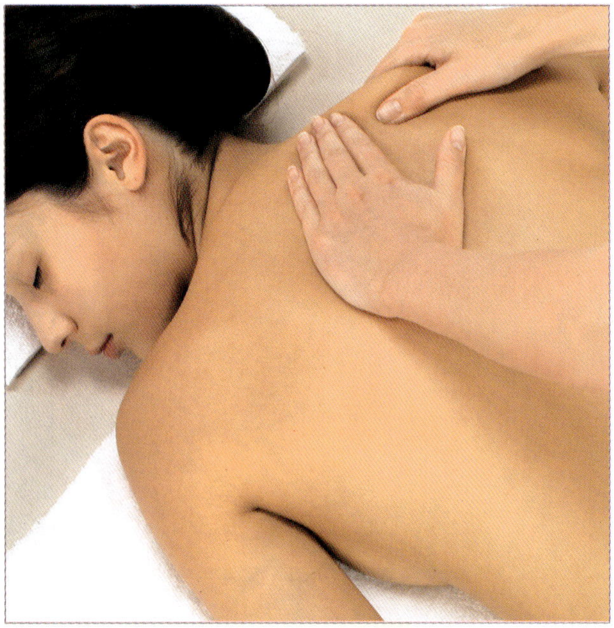

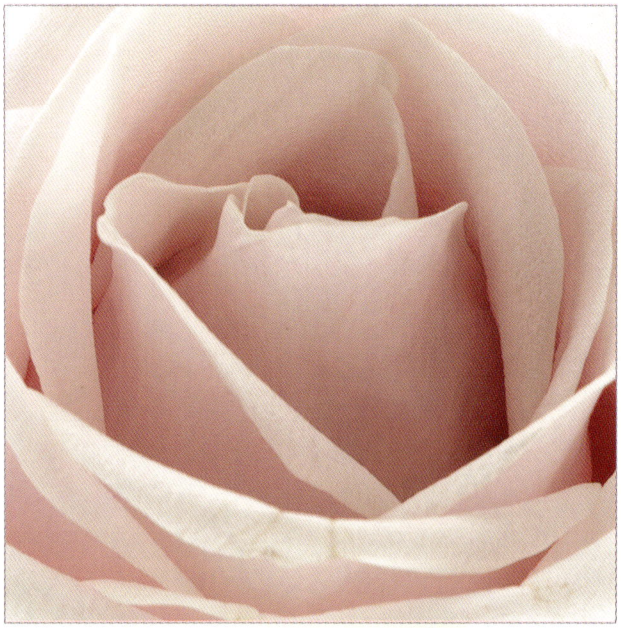

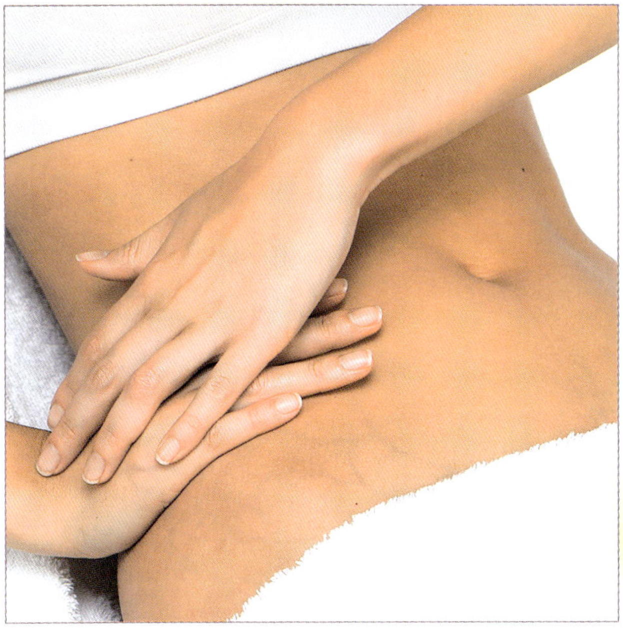

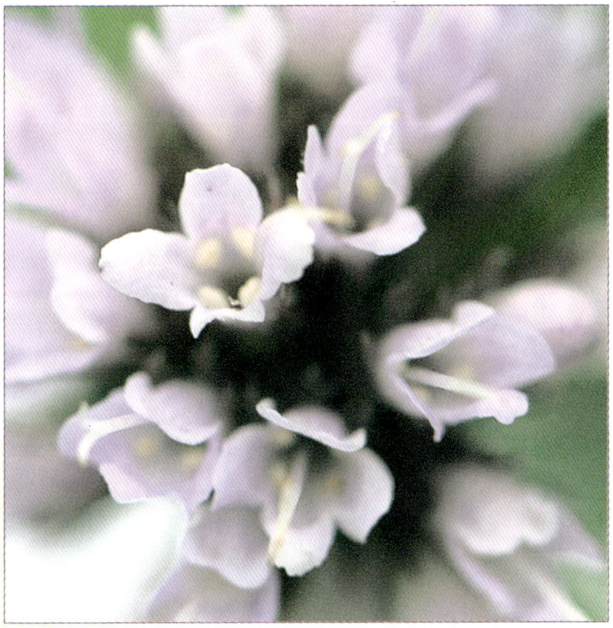

# foreword

Having worked with essential oils for some 35 years, I am still amazed at their power to heal and uplift. There is no other modality in which touch, smell and plant medicine coincide so perfectly. It fascinates me, for example, that peppermint oil can relieve tension headaches, aid digestion, and invigorate the mind so effectively. Also, microbiological research has revealed why tea tree oil is so useful in treating infectious conditions such as athlete's foot and acne. These are not whimsical claims, there is good clinical evidence supporting each of these properties.

Essential oils can be useful in many ways, and this beautifully designed book contains a feast of information about them, including many valuable safety tips which I urge you to follow carefully. Skin reactions to essential oils are probably the most common "side-effect" from aromatherapy, and the higher the concentration of essential oil, the more likely a reaction will occur. So please be sure to follow Jennie's directions for diluting and using these wonderful healing oils.

I have known Jennie for many years, first as an aromatherapy student, and then as a teacher at the Tisserand Institute, and so it is gratifying to see her evolve into such a capable writer. Like many people, Jennie has a passion for plants and essential oils, and she writes with both vitality and wisdom. I think I can appreciate how much work has gone into researching the history and tradition of each plant, and into creating the hundreds of blends in this book. Jennie's breadth of knowledge and many years of experience are showcased here in this wonderful introduction to aromatherapy and massage. Enjoy.

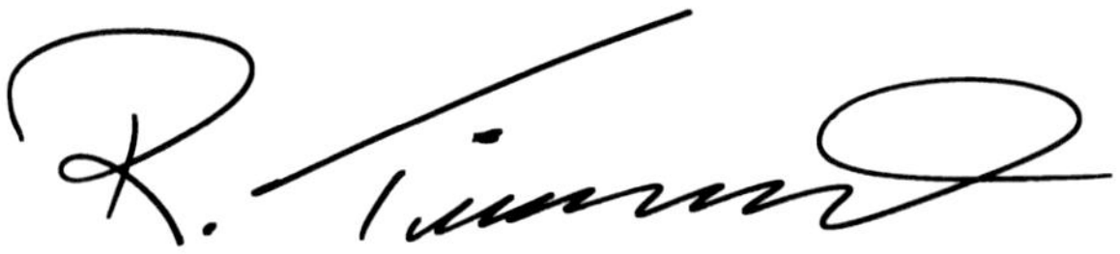

# author's introduction

In my parents' first photo album of me as a child there is a picture that always makes me smile. I am toddling in the park with my mother, in the sunshine, and stooping over some flowers, examining them with intense interest. I have always been fascinated by flowers, especially roses. I also know that when I was little my enthusiasm for their smell landed me in bushes and covered me with scratches on more than one occasion! I sometimes wonder if I was always meant to end up working as an aromatherapist because I have always loved the fragrances of plants thanks to my keen sense of smell. It was, however, many years before I knew anything about aromatherapy – my education and early career took me in a very different direction, into marketing and the corporate world.

I first came across aromatherapy about sixteen years ago when I went into a health food shop for no particular reason and saw some odd little bottles on a shelf. I asked what they were and was told "essential oils". I had no idea what this meant, but I bought some lavender oil – which I instantly adored – and a book: Robert Tisserand's *Art of Aromatherapy*. I read it from cover to cover. I had always been interested in aromatic plants and knew they were used in herbal medicine, but the idea of using natural fragrances – essential oils – as a therapy was a new and intriguing idea to me.

Because I am the kind of person who always likes to find out more about things, I decided I had to go and learn aromatherapy. My teacher, Robert Tisserand himself, was instrumental in guiding and developing my passion for the fragrances of essential oils. From the very beginning, I realized that aromatherapy is powerful, yet subtle. I came to understand that the marriage of essential oils and massage is crucial to the experience of relaxation which is at the heart of this caring therapy. Together, they bring a sense of deep peace and calm to the recipient, allowing the body and mind to rest. This is the most important aspect, to me, of the therapy I have practised and taught for so long. In this state of relaxation the body can rebalance and restore itself.

Over the years I have given aromatherapy massage to many people, and have seen again and again how the benefits of touch and aroma help to create a window of calm in times of stress. Whether tension arises through mental, emotional or physical causes, the gentle art of aromatherapy can change the tempo of life, teaching in a silent and subtle way the lesson of slower rhythms. Some stress is good for us, to be sure, but modern living is generally conducted at a mad pace with very little opportunity for slowing down. Aromatherapy massage can be a very useful tool to relieve anxiety as well as to release the deeper-rooted aches and pains caused by stress.

In the time I have been working as an aromatherapist there has been a huge increase in interest in aromatherapy generally. From being an approach that was considered very "on the fringe" when I began, aromatherapy is now being used in settings such as hospitals, doctors' surgeries and hospices, and homes for older people or those in mental health care; the benefits of touch and aroma bring deep relaxation, improve sleep and improve communication. Some businesses vaporize essential oils in the work environment – in Japan they say it increases concentration and productivity – or have massage therapists working on the staff. Aromatherapy is developing into an approach with wide applications and is full of future potential.

However, as well as these developments we do see the cosmetics industry flooding the market with thousands of aromatherapy products – toothpastes,

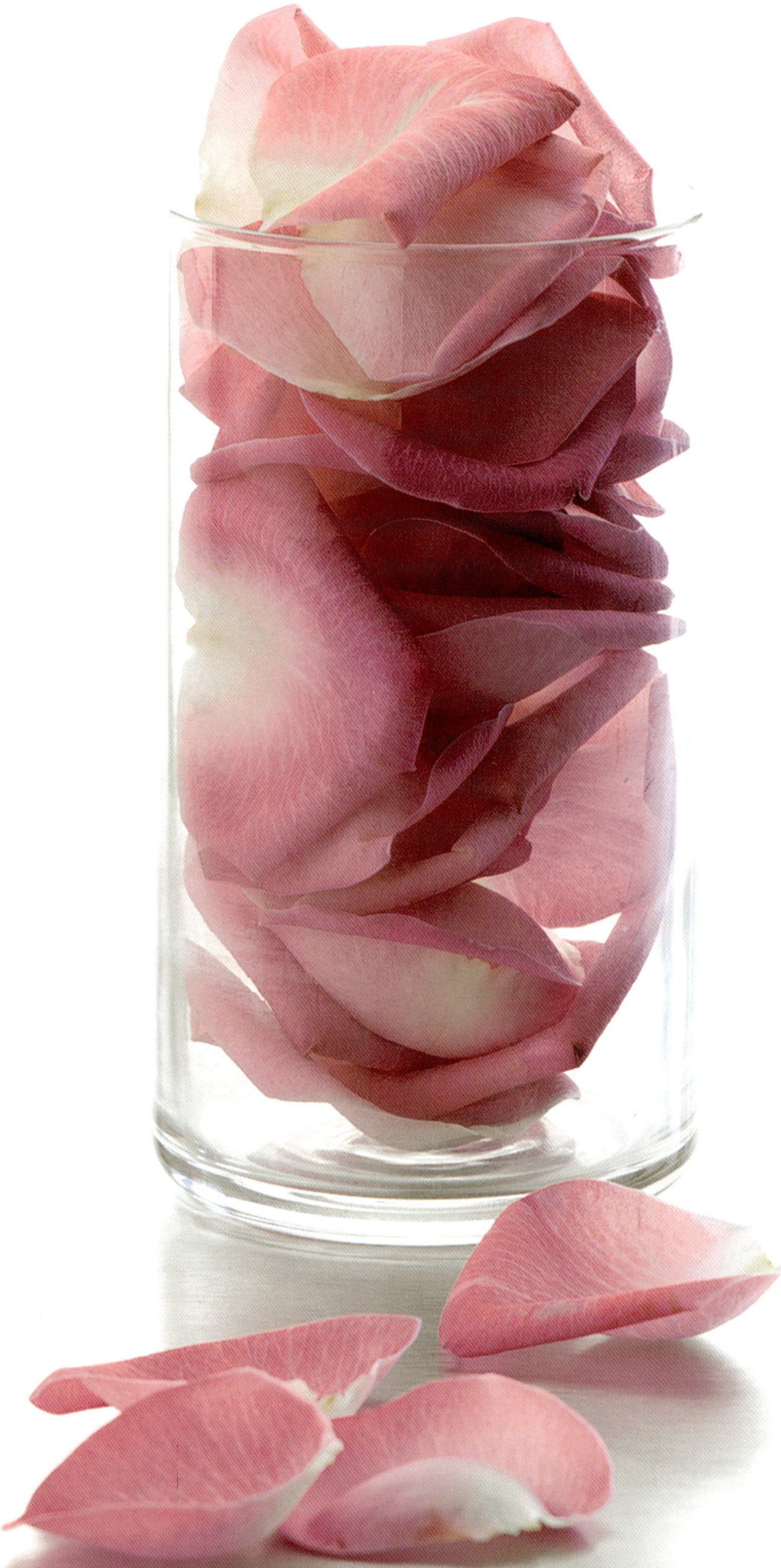

shower gels, shampoos, face creams to name but a few. This means that there is a much wider awareness of the word "aromatherapy" than when I came into the field years ago, but I believe the real meaning of the therapy is in danger of becoming diluted. True aromatherapy is a skill, both in the art of creating blends of essential oils and in applying them. This takes time to develop and practise – there are many different techniques that can be used to apply massage and essential oils. If you are prepared to spend the time, the results will be worth the effort – and you are learning something that will be of real value to you in your life.

This book will help you to learn the skill of applying aromatherapy to yourself and those around you in a way that is safe, beneficial and in-keeping with the principles of the therapy. Through learning the techniques of simple massage and understanding the uses of many different essential oils, you can begin to use aromatherapy in daily life and feel real benefits – such as better sleep patterns, fewer aches and pains, improved skin condition and restored energy levels. Aromatherapy is a tool, and if used safely and appropriately it helps to improve physical, mental and emotional well-being as well as create a caring and nurturing environment.

I have practised and taught aromatherapy for the past 13 years and in that time my love of the oils has deepened through a growing interest in cultivating aromatic plants myself. I am keen to explain the benefits of aromatherapy because I have spent so many years using it on clients, my family and myself, and experiencing the difference it can make. This book is designed to bring together touch and aroma, massage and essential oils, so that anyone can begin to experience the wonderful benefits of aromatherapy. As you learn more about oils and how to apply them, I hope this will be the beginning of a long and fruitful journey of self-discovery for you, as it has been and continues to be for me.

# how to use this book

Welcome to *Aromatherapy Massage for You* – a practical manual which shows you how to use aromatherapy techniques safely on yourself and other people. In this busy day and age, aromatherapy can be used as a valuable tool to relieve stress and improve health and well-being. This book will guide you through all the steps you need to start working with aromatherapy yourself.

Aromatherapy uses natural fragrances – essential oils – taken from many different plants, and, as such, has become a highly popular form of natural health care. Essential oils smell delightful and by combining them in different ways you can create wonderful natural fragrances. However, it is vitally important to understand them and use them safely. Giving you the information with which to do this is one of the main purposes of this book. Aromatherapy is also fun and creative; you will find many different blends of essential oils to make, all with detailed instructions, so you will be able to try out and experience the effects of essential oils yourself.

Massage is the most effective way of delivering aromatherapy; it is a form of therapeutic touch which should be nurturing, respectful and pleasant to receive. This book will show you many different massage techniques that are simple and effective, and will discuss important massage issues such as safety and working with care. If you have never tried to massage anyone before, don't worry – this book will show you how to go about it. There are short step-by-step routines for massaging different areas of the body, which you can combine to make longer massage treatments. You can also practise aromatherapy on yourself, and you will find some suggested routines for this too.

In *Aromatherapy Massage for You* there are three main chapters to discover; the first is a detailed exploration of the world of aromatherapy and essential oils, full of fascinating facts and details about these natural aromas, where they come from and how they are obtained. The second is a practical chapter, which shows you basic massage strokes and routines, accompanied by a variety of suggested blends for each one. The third chapter is a directory of 48 essential oils, some more common and some more unusual, which you can use as a guide as you start to collect oils for your own use. You will find detailed information on how to use each oil along with safety guidelines and more blends to try.

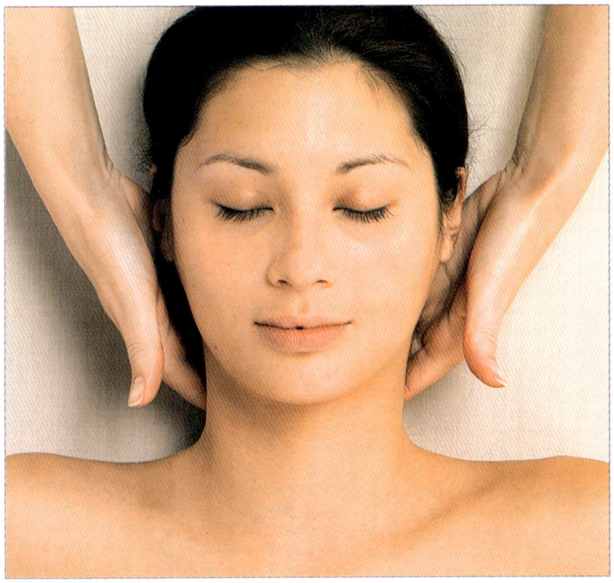

Aromatherapy can make a real difference to your life; the more you use it, the more you will realize its effects. Better sleep, deeper relaxation, help with aches and pains, increased mental clarity and a sense of inner peace are just some of the benefits. There is also the satisfaction of helping someone else – they may simply feel more relaxed or may gain relief from aches, pains or emotional stress. As you learn aromatherapy I hope it will become a wonderful caring tool in your hands and that this book will be a valuable guide and help to you.

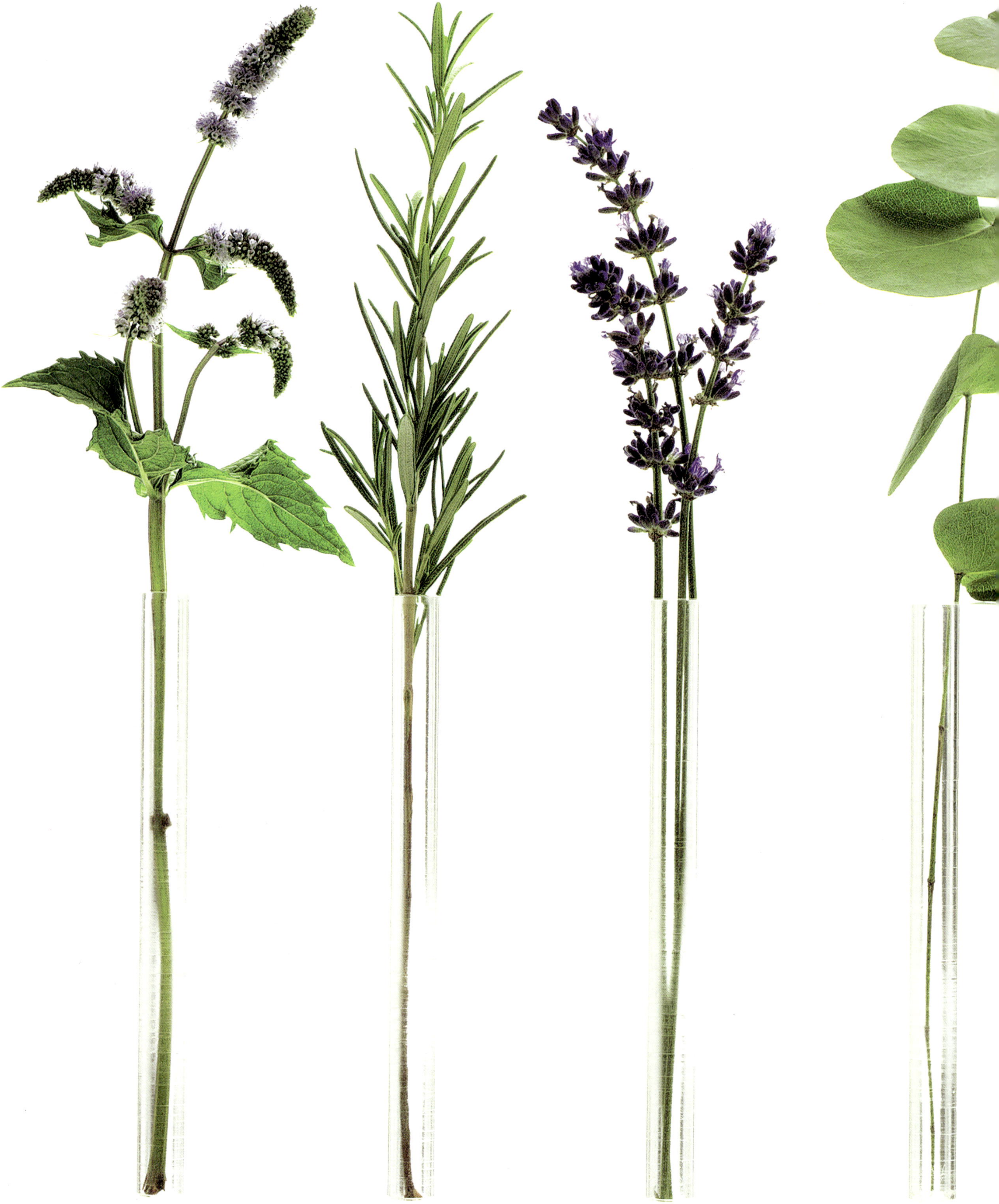

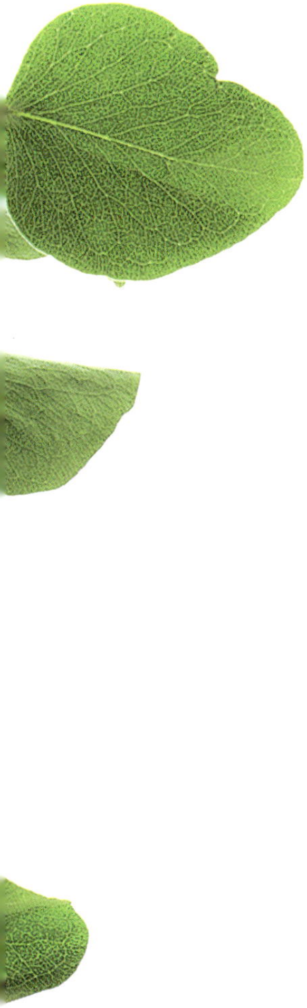

CHAPTER ONE

# touch and fragrance

*Aromatherapy massage links together two highly important senses – touch and smell. It combines the caring and beneficial touch of massage with the distinctive aromas of essential oil blends, which reach the mind and influence mood and feelings to create a unique therapeutic experience.*

In this chapter we explore the world of aromatherapy from its ancient origins to modern times, and learn about the core principles that apply to this holistic therapy. We examine in more detail the powerful positive effects that aromatherapy massage can have on the body and mind, and discover how this works, through the amazing organ of the skin and the sense of smell. Information is presented about the vital essential oils themselves; where they come from, theories on why they exist, and the methods by which they are extracted. I also offer some detailed guidelines on the safe use of essential oils, which are designed to encourage you to practise aromatherapy with confidence, and advice on the purchase and storage of oils, as well as practical information on how to make up your aromatherapy blends.

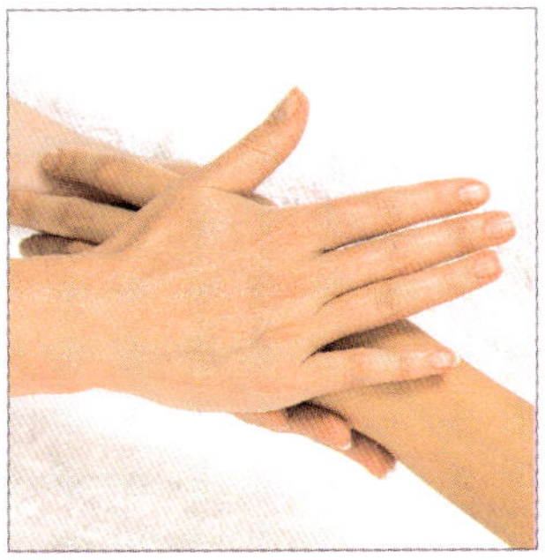

# the story of aromatherapy

Aromatherapy has its roots in antiquity, but the word itself is a 20th-century invention. The use of aromatic plants as medicines, incense and cosmetics in ancient times is well-documented, and over the centuries this led to the development of aromatherapy and its use of essential oils from these plants as a healing tool in our lives today.

Modern techniques of distillation and extraction now enable many countries to produce essential oils and export them across the globe. Indeed, part of the attraction of an aromatherapy blend of oils lies in combining exotic plant extracts from different locations in a single mixture. Yet, the perfuming of a carrier oil with different fragrances is definitely nothing new.

**AROMATICS IN THE PAST**

The word "perfume" comes from the Latin *per fumum* which means "by smoke". This reflects the original use of aromatic plants as incense, burned on altars as a means of communication with the spirit world. The ancient Chinese had a great love of incense, burning extracts of plants such as cassia, cinnamon and sandalwood; and historical evidence suggests that the Hindu culture in India absorbed this tradition from China around 5,000 years ago, adding such aromatics as frankincense, benzoin gum and jasmine. The Hindu god Shiva was traditionally worshipped with incense every four hours, day and night.

The use of aromatics spread to Ancient Egypt, where the aroma of incense in ritual became a crucial way of identifying the presence of the divine. The ancient Egyptians soaked aromatic gums, roots and herbs in oil or pressed them into trays of animal fat and laid them in the sun, creating "unguents", highly perfumed fatty ointments, which they then used as cosmetics and as fragrance. The tomb of Tutankhamun contained many fine alabaster jars filled with unguents, perfumed with myrrh, frankincense, cassia and other expensive ingredients. The Pharaoh lived in fragrance – his clothes were perfumed, his body anointed daily, his living environment filled with constant aromatic reminders of his semi-divine nature. Even after death, his body cavities were filled with preservative aromatic gums and spices to ensure he would reach the afterlife in perfect condition.

This extensive use of aromatics spread from Egypt to the Greek and Roman worlds, and is recorded in the famous *Herbal* of Pedanius Dioscorides, a physician in the service of the Roman Emperor Tiberius, who wrote down the identity and use of all the medicinal and aromatic plants known in the first century CE. Between the seventh and 13th centuries, the Arab world became renowned for its use of herbs, spices, gums and roots in the treatment of disease. Notably, the physician and scholar Abu-Ibn-Sina (980–1037), often known as Avicenna, is credited with inventing a form of distillation which was used to extract essential oils and aromatic water; roses being among the first flowers to be used.

During the Middle Ages in Europe, aromatic herbs had a variety of uses. They were mixed with floor rushes to try to disguise odours, and were brewed into teas, infusions or washes to fight infection. Lavender, rosemary, sage and thyme were particularly popular. By the 16th century, distillation equipment made the extraction of essential oils from aromatic plants more efficient, and the oils were supplied as remedies by apothecaries. In the 17th century, during the Great Plague in London, physicians wore masks with protruding beaks filled with spices and herbs to protect themselves from infection. In effect, essential oils and aromatics were being used as antiseptics, but without a direct undertanding of why or how they actually worked.

During the 17th and 18th centuries in Europe, divisions appeared in what had previously been a virtually seamless use of aromatics in medicine, ritual and cosmetics. The perfumery industry, particularly in France, moved toward producing fragrances for toiletry purposes; then apothecaries who used herbal remedies split from physicians who were becoming interested in the first synthetic drugs, the origins of the modern drug industry. By the 19th and 20th centuries, the production of essential oils had declined and their use was largely limited to perfumery and cosmetics, and as flavourings in food.

## AROMATHERAPY IN THE MODERN WORLD

The term "aromatherapy" was invented in the early 20th century by French perfume chemist René Gattefosse, who had used lavendar essential oil to treat a severe burn he received in a laboratory accident. Gattefosse found that the oil had a remarkable healing effect on his injury, even preventing scarring. In 1937 he published a book, *Aromathérapie*, in which he proposed that essential oils, far from being mere fragrance ingredients, could also have dramatic healing potential. His book discussed many aspects of essential oil use, particularly wound-healing. Another Frenchman, Dr Jean Valnet, took the approach further and used essential oils in wound care, as antiviral agents, and as anti-rheumatic and pain-relieving tools. He saw aromatherapy as a bridge between the experience-based herbal traditions of the past and the modern drug culture. In France today doctors continue to follow Dr Valnet's methods, using essential oils in a medical context as natural antimicrobial agents. His own book, also called *Aromathérapie* and published in 1964, is still regarded as a classic.

Also in France in the early 1960s, bio-chemist Marguerite Maury applied Dr Valnet's approach to beauty therapy; she created the notion of an "individual prescription" or blend of essential oils tailored to suit the client's specific needs, applied mainly by massage. Maury's book, *The Secret of Life and Youth*, delved into the psychological effects of smell on the mind, something that would become a key factor in the development of aromatherapy as we practise it today. When renowned aromatherapist Robert Tisserand published his first book on the subject, *The Art of Aromatherapy*, in 1977, the notion of essential oils as physically and psychologically supportive tools was firmly established, with massage as the key method of application. It is this principle that has shaped the growth of aromatherapy in modern times, into one of the most popular of all the so-called "complementary therapies".

Why is aromatherapy so popular? Tisserand called it "feel-good therapy", which it certainly is; the deep sense of relaxation and well-being produced by treatment is the reason people enjoy it so much, and the aromas of the oils have such uplifting effects on mood. It is also a link back to nature at a time when many people have very little actual contact with the earth; ironically, it is our so-called "primitive" sense, the sense of smell, that is stimulated by this therapy. By-passing our ever-busy minds, the deeper feelings evoked by essential oils bring rejuvenation and restoration to body and spirit.

# principles of aromatherapy

Aromatherapy is a tool that we can use for many purposes. As you begin to explore the practice in more depth, it will help to have an understanding of some of the underlying core principles that give aromatherapy a framework.

Aromatherapy is known as a "complementary therapy", that is to say an approach to health and well-being that complements conventional medicine. Even as a lay person practising aromatherapy on only family and friends, you are working in a healing context, and every healing method is founded on a set of principles that underpin the practise of the skill. Modern aromatherapy and, in particular, aromatherapy massage, is based on the following ideas, which are all interconnected.

**HOLISM**

The word "holism" is derived from the word "whole", meaning complete or entire. It is also connected to the old Germanic word *hael* which means holy and healthy (as in "hale and hearty"). Holism means, simply, that the health of the whole person is taken into account, not just their isolated symptoms. The aim is to balance a person's entire system – in therapeutic terms, this is seen as mind, body and spirit being in harmony. This is nothing new. Only in the West have we become accustomed to separating treatment of the body from that of the mind and spirit. In the East such ideas have continued in an unbroken line from early civilization to this day. For example, the Indian Vedic tradition describes the physical body as inextricably linked to the energetic map of the body called the chakra system, which allows the energy of spirit to take form in matter. Also, the Far Eastern medical traditions of China and Japan describe vital energy flowing through the body along channels called meridians, just beyond the physical body but inextricably linked to it. By manipulating the flow of this energy, through such approaches as shiatsu or acupuncture, the body rebalances itself.

As a healing tool combining both touch and smell, or the physical and the non-physical, aromatherapy massage sits well in the holistic framework. The individual blends of oils mixed for the recipient's treatment are chosen to complement the person's physical and emotional state. Massage is the means of application, but, much more than that, it allows the giving of a caring and soothing touch, which helps to de-stress the system completely and sends deep messages of calm to the mind. In today's frantic world, this is a vital need. Many physical and emotional illnesses are the result of the human system being stressed to breaking point. The simple act of aromatherapy massage can help to rebalance and rejuvenate body, mind and spirit.

**HEALING**

Aromatherapy is also a form of healing. What is healing? It can be described as a positive change of some kind which restores balance to a system that is over- or under-performing in some way. One of the main reasons that a particular health problem occurs is because the body is reacting to an area of stress somewhere within its system. Conventional medicine chooses to focus on the problem itself, sometimes with very direct interventions, and these can be vital for extreme situations such as surgical emergencies or acute problems such as a heart attack. The complementary therapies, including aromatherapy massage, concentrate on the terrain of the body system itself, with the idea that, if at all possible, prevention is better than cure. Aromatherapy massage works well as a supportive treatment for chronic problems, which unfold over a long period of time. Essential oils and massage, sensitively given, can gently allow the body to rebalance itself, which it is very capable of doing. We inhabit bodies and minds with extremely sensitive capabilities especially when it comes to adapting to new situations, and our bodies are capable of amazing feats of repair and renewal right down to the cellular level, especially when they achieve a relaxed, restful state.

Healing is the point where a change occurs to bring us back to harmony. Often my clients in the treatment setting have said that taking time out from the craziness of life, and experiencing a calm environment and the effects of aromatherapy massage, immediately shows how much they need that change.

## HEALTH

Another word connected to the old Germanic *hael*, health is much more than the absence of illness. It is a state in which you are in balance; your mind is clear and your emotions at peace; you are in tune with your environment and feel nourished by your surroundings as well as by the people with whom you live. This probably sounds impossible to achieve, but more and more people are beginning to acknowledge the importance of trying to realize this goal. All the money and status in the world is worth nothing if getting it makes you too sick to enjoy it. Sometimes it takes a real crisis in body or mind to bring the need for a change of attitude to the fore. Indeed, many of my clients have spoken to me of the way in which illness has been a great teacher, showing the need for a fresh appraisal of what is truly important in life.

Using aromatherapy massage can be the start of a change in lifestyle; the more aromatherapy finds its way into your everyday life, the more you will start to pay attention to aspects such as diet, relaxation, exercise and creativity. These are all parts of achieving a holistic approach to health. Aromatherapy massage is, above all, an experience that re-awakens senses that are often dulled. Our senses are an amazing interface with our external environment; waking them up is a great way to begin to improve our health and well-being.

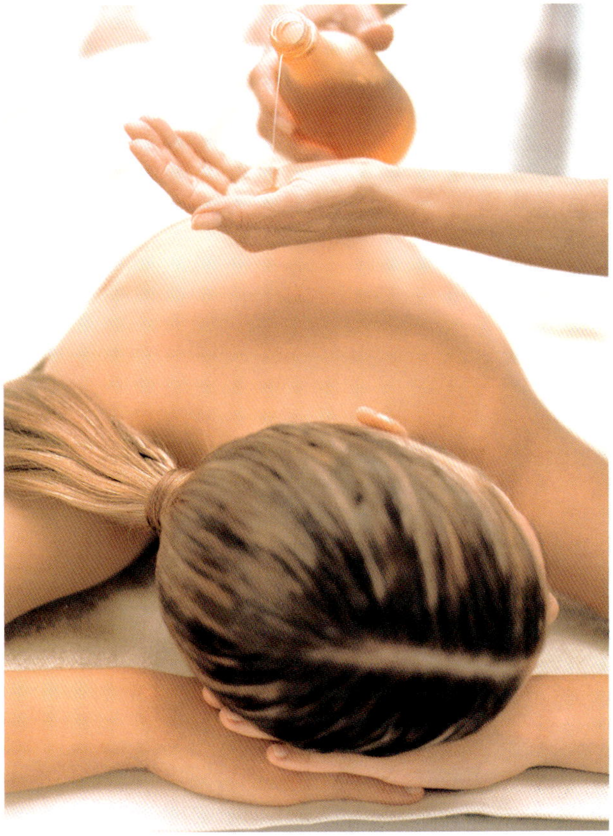

# what is an essential oil?

Essential oils are highly concentrated fragrances that are found in aromatic plants. These plants make up a mere one per cent of all plant species on earth, yet this tiny proportion includes plant families that human beings have used for thousands years in cooking, medicine, ritual and cosmetics.

A common example of an aromatic plant family is Labiatae (Lamiaceae), which includes the Mediterranean herbs thyme, rosemary, marjoram, melissa, sage, lavender, peppermint and oregano. Approximately half of all essential oils used in aromatherapy come from this family group. Two further plant families provide many of the remaining oils commonly used in aromatherapy. These are the Rutaceae group, which includes all the citrus fruits, and the Umbelliferae family, which includes angelica, fennel, coriander, carrot and parsley.

Essential oils are found in different parts of plants: in the Labiatae group the strongest fragrance is often found in the leaves. In the Rutaceae group the peel of citrus fruit is packed full of tiny essential oil sacs – if you pare off a fine strip of peel from a lemon and turn it over, you will see them all quite clearly. Plants from the Umbelliferae family contain essential oil in their leaves, stalks and pungent seeds. Other locations for fragrance in plants are flowers, woods, resins and roots.

## PLANT PROCESSES

Exactly why essential oils are present in these plants is a question that still perplexes botanists. There are different theories, ranging from seeing the oils as simple waste products to viewing them as specialist substances, which give the plant an evolutionary edge in a highly competitive natural world. Essential oils in flowers are responsible for the sweet aromas that attract insects to come and pollinate the bloom at its peak. In leaves, the essential oils help to maintain a flat and shiny surface, which keeps the leaf open and unshrivelled even in high temperatures, in turn allowing the plant to keep breathing and producing food. Essential oils in woody branches, tree trunks or roots have insect-repellant properties, and aromatic seeds attract birds and other animals to feed; their hard cases pass unharmed through the digestive tracts of these creatures and fall to the ground in droppings to germinate and reproduce away from their original location.

## GEOGRAPHY AND ENVIRONMENT

Plants containing essential oils exist all over the globe. Many come from temperate latitudes; plants such as lavender, peppermint, rose and orange live across continental Europe, from France and Germany in the north, stretching as far south as the Mediterranean Sea. North Africa and the Middle East produce plant oils that form the key ingredients of many ancient perfumes – frankincense, myrrh, cassia and cedarwood. Heady, exotic-smelling oils, such as nutmeg, patchouli, sandalwood, lemongrass and cinnamon, come from plants found in tropical locations including India, Indonesia and China. Australia and New Zealand are the producers of the strong antibacterial oils found in tea tree, manuka, kanuka and eucalyptus. South America produces much rosewood and orange oil; and the islands of Madagascar and Réunion in the Indian Ocean are major producers of ylang ylang and vetiver.

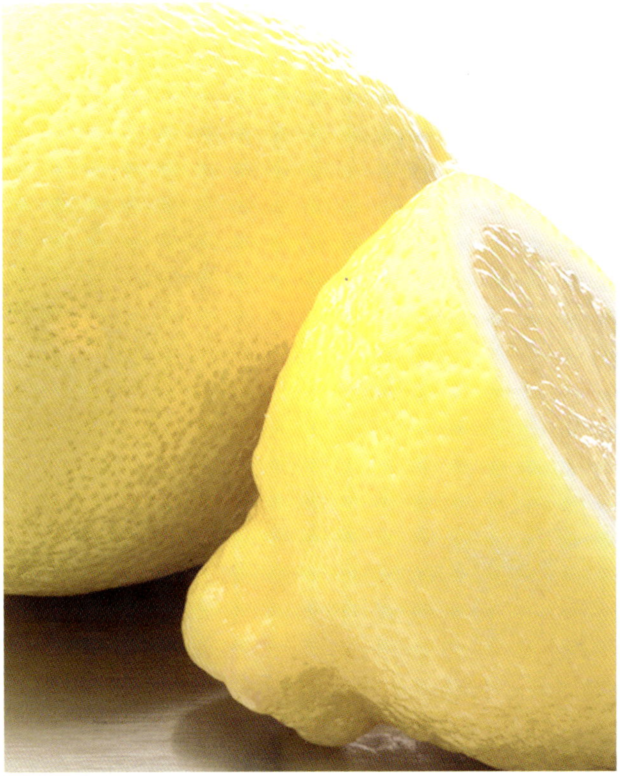

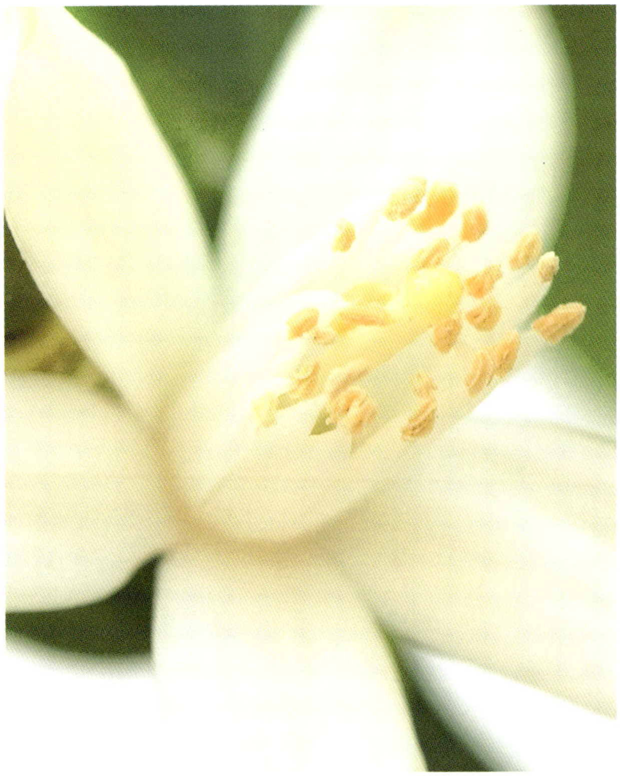

## EXTRACTION METHODS

Most essential oils are obtained by steam distillation. This requires a great deal of plant material – for example, it takes approximately 0.75 tonnes of lavender or rosemary to produce one litre (2 pints) of essential oil – and commercial extraction relies on farms to produce large quantities of the plants. In the case of rose essential oil, it takes around one hundred blooms to generate just one drop of essential oil, which is the reason why this oil is so expensive. Growers have to know the optimum time to harvest crops to obtain the best quality and maximum amount of essential oil. This may vary each year because of changes in weather patterns and the length of season; and such factors produce slight variations, year on year, in the aroma of essential oils.

For distillation, plant material is packed into a large metal container called a still, before steam is pumped through at pressure. This lifts the aromatic molecules from the plant fibre; the aromatic steam passes through a cooling pipe and changes, or condenses, back into water, with the essential oil floating on the surface. This is then siphoned off. The remaining water is also aromatic and useful; it is called a "hydrolat". Lavender, rose, and orange flower water are commonly used as simple skin toners or even in cooking.

Delicate flowers such as jasmine cannot be processed with distillation as it would destroy the petals. Instead, these flowers are soaked in chemical solvent and then processed to give a product called an absolute – a thick and highly fragranced liquid. In aromatherapy, jasmine absolute is the most commonly used; many other exotic absolutes, such as narcissus or mimosa, are used in the formulation of fine perfumes.

Citrus oils are obtained by expression, or squeezing, the essential oil out of the peel of oranges, lemons, grapefruits or mandarins. These oils are fresh and zesty, and add light and uplifting notes to massage blends.

# aromatherapy and the mind

The word "aromatherapy" implies that we can achieve some kind of therapeutic effect simply as a result of the use of fragrance. "Smell-therapy" might seem like an unusual idea, but, in fact, aromas can have powerful effects on the mind, mood and feelings.

Passing a rose bush in full bloom on a warm summer's evening, you might feel compelled to stop and inhale the scent of the flowers – almost forgetting where you are. Walking in a pine forest might make you take big, deep breaths – the fresh, resiny scent of the trees giving you a feeling of space and well-being. And the warm smell of cakes or bread may conjure up feelings of security and homeliness. We react to smells almost without realizing it, and sometimes those reactions can change our patterns of thought and behaviour.

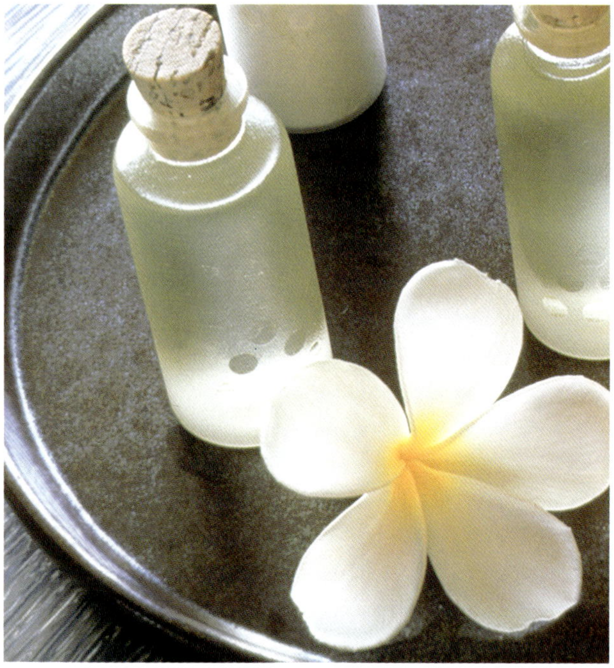

**HOW DOES THE SENSE OF SMELL WORK?**

The anatomical story of the sense of smell is closely tied to the brain. The structures associated with smell begin outside the head with the nose itself, and the nostrils, which allow air to circulate upward. As we inhale we bring scented molecules up the passageways of the nostrils to the back of the nose. Here they are trapped at a microscopic level in patches of cells called olfactory receptors; these trigger tiny electrical impulses into the olfactory bulbs, which act as relay stations deeper in the head. Stronger impulses carry the message of the sense of smell along olfactory nerves, into the core of the brain itself. This whole process takes less than two seconds.

The sense of smell is interpreted in different brain areas. If a smell reaches the deep inner area (the limbic system) the response may be non-verbal – perhaps a sound like "mmm", or a strong emotional response of like or dislike, not expressed in words, but through facial expressions or a change in posture. If the smell impulse reaches the grey matter in the brain's neo-cortex, it may link it to events, places, memories or feelings and cause these to be verbally expressed, perhaps with some analysis. Either way, it is difficult to avoid reacting to smell stimuli. As well as these noticeable brain responses, the body may produce saliva if there is an association with food, or deepen the breathing and calm the pulse if the aroma is perceived as relaxing.

## AROMATHERAPY AS MIND–BODY COMMUNICATION

Using essential oils enables highly concentrated natural aromas to come into contact with the nose and brain. As the aroma travels up the nose toward the receptors, we will immediately experience certain responses. The most common sign is a deep sigh, as the pressures of the day fall away. Smells of nature have associations with space, time away from cares, perhaps places people have visited or memories from childhood. The effect of such impressions can deeply enhance the effects of massage, which gets to work on physical tensions and aches; as the brain relaxes, it communicates relaxation to the body.

I once gave a massage to a client who had been recently bereaved, and who talked about the illness that had left her mother so weak and helpless. She had been relieved when her mother passed away, but felt some guilt about this. When she smelled the aroma of rose essential oil, her face changed, her eyes closed and a flush came over her cheeks. She opened her eyes after a moment and said she could see her mother as she had been; someone who had loved flowers and taken pride in her garden. This was the beginning of her own healing.

Associations with smells are highly individual and there are no set rules. When choosing oils for a blend, a simple guideline is to check that the recipient likes the aromas, individually and in combination. This is a very important part of aromatherapy; if the person dislikes the smells, they may have strong negative reactions and relaxation is almost impossible to achieve. The weather, the season, or someone's mood or level of mental activity can also affect preferences. Aromatherapy uses fragrances from plants – scents of nature. Just as our environment changes on a daily basis, so does the balance between our mind and our body; aromatherapy can help to keep our mental processes fresh and responsive.

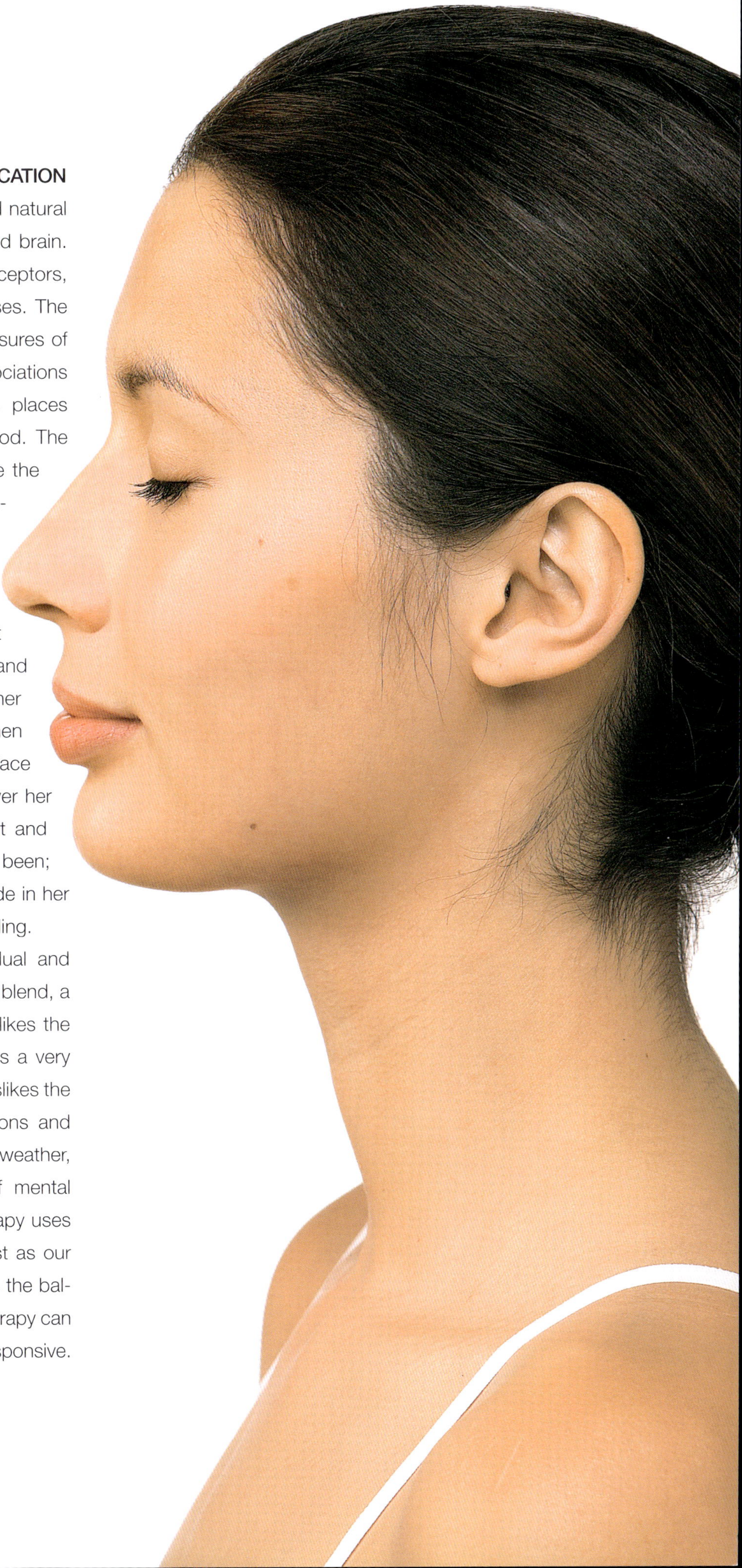

# aromatherapy and the body

Essential oils come into contact with the physical body through the vegetable carrier oil that is used as a base for the blend. This blend is then applied using massage, so that the muscles and soft tissue benefit from the massage strokes, while the essential oils penetrate the body through the large area of the skin.

Massage is one of the most important ways in which to use essential oils, although there are other methods of employing them, such as in baths, inhalations or vaporizers. However, the main advantage of a body massage treatment is that it massages in the blend over as extensive an area as possible; this achieves maximum absorption in a very gentle and diluted way.

**SKIN ABSORPTION**

The skin is a complex organ; it provides protection for the body, regulates temperature, and allows toxins to be released through sweat glands. Richly supplied with tiny blood vessels, it is also full of nerve endings which are responsible for relaying the experience of touch to the brain. Our skin is a direct interface with the outside world and our actual environment – whether this is hot, cold, wet, dry, sharp, soft, rough or smooth. Our daily lives are governed by touch, by everything with which we come into contact, whether alive or inert.

The skin has several important layers. First, the epidermis, the outer layer that we see, is made of millions of cells which overlap each other like microscopic roofing tiles. These provide a semi-permeable barrier which allows moisture and toxins to escape, but does not allow too much water to be absorbed. These epidermal cells are constantly rising to the surface and

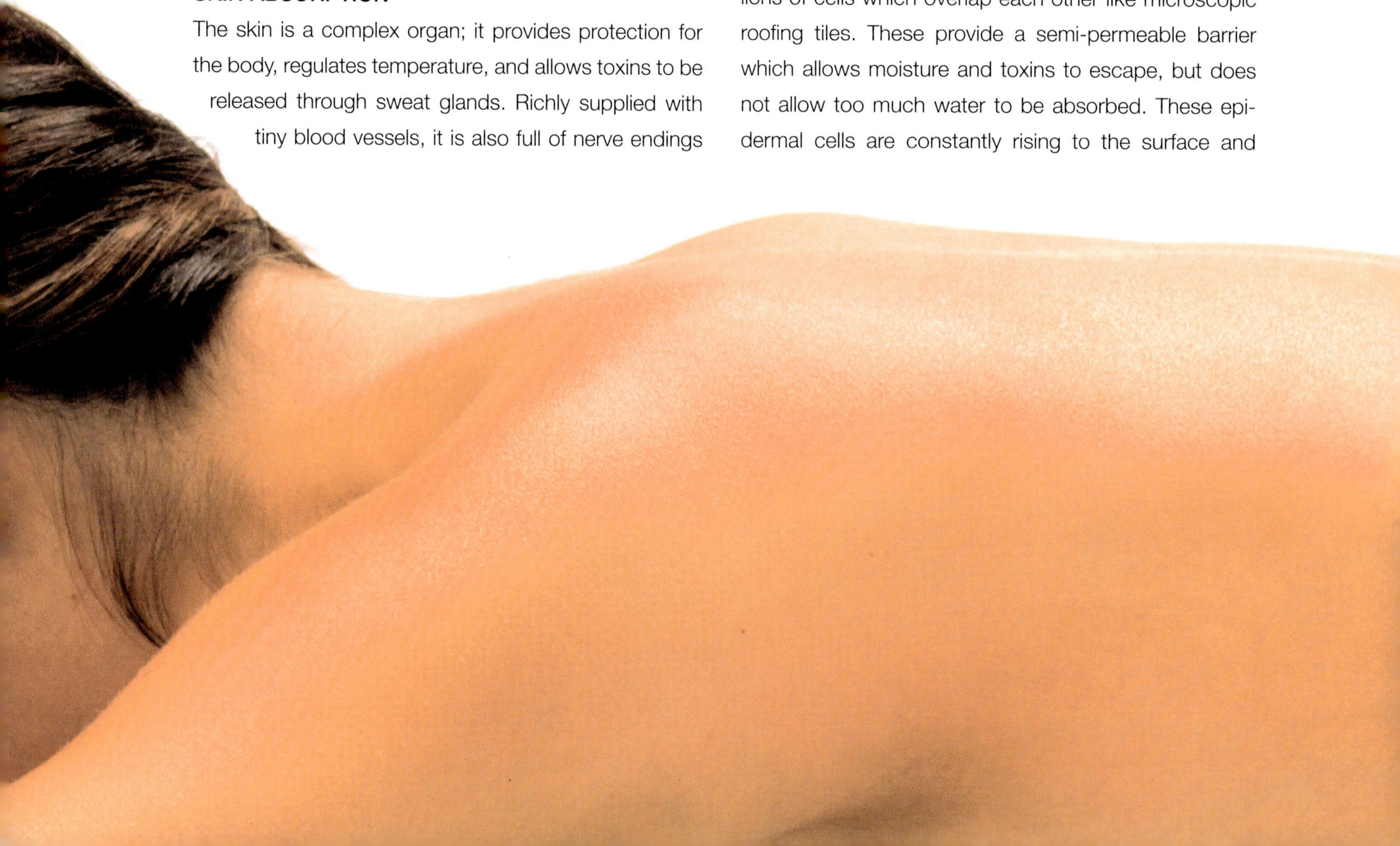

being replaced as old ones get rubbed off by clothing, or by washing and drying the skin. They contain the protein keratin, which is also found in the hair and nails.

The middle layer of the skin is called the dermis. It is made up of blood vessels, nerve endings, sweat glands and sebaceous glands (which secrete sebum, the skin's own natural oil, onto the epidermis to keep it supple). This layer is where nutrients are delivered to the skin via the blood vessels, and waste products taken away. Beneath the dermis lies a third layer, of subcutaneous fat, which is where all our hair follicles have their roots.

When we apply an aromatherapy blend to the skin, the vegetable carrier oil stays in the upper epidermal layer, helping to moisturize the outer surface of the skin. This is because the molecules in the carrier oil are too big to be absorbed any deeper. Essential oils also have highly beneficial effects on the upper skin surface but, because they contain much smaller molecules, they are also absorbed through the epidermis, down into the dermal layer and into the thin blood vessels just under the skin. From here they are carried into the circulation. For more information on the specific properties of individual essential oils and blends, see the oil profiles in Chapter 3; pp.86–139.

**RESPIRATORY EFFECTS**

A full-body aromatherapy massage treatment typically lasts for one hour, so that the person being treated spends a long time inhaling the fragrance of the blend used. As well as the psychological benefits of this (see pp.20–21), essential oil molecules can travel into the respiratory system and cause a deepening of the breath as the airways open or dilate, and the lungs inflate to a fuller capacity than normal. Breath is vital to life, and deep breathing has many beneficial effects – it improves the experience of relaxation, nourishes cells with oxygen, and improves vitality and well-being.

**EXCRETION PATHWAYS**

Once essential oils are in the circulatory system, they will travel around the body for several hours before being excreted, mainly via the kidneys, but also in sweat or, in tiny amounts, in the breath. We can see how quickly essential oils can travel through the system by using the strong aroma of garlic. If a clove is cut in half and rubbed on the soles of the feet, the odour of garlic will come out in the breath an hour or so later! Some essential oil compounds stay longer in the system, but the amounts are very tiny and are eventually excreted by the body.

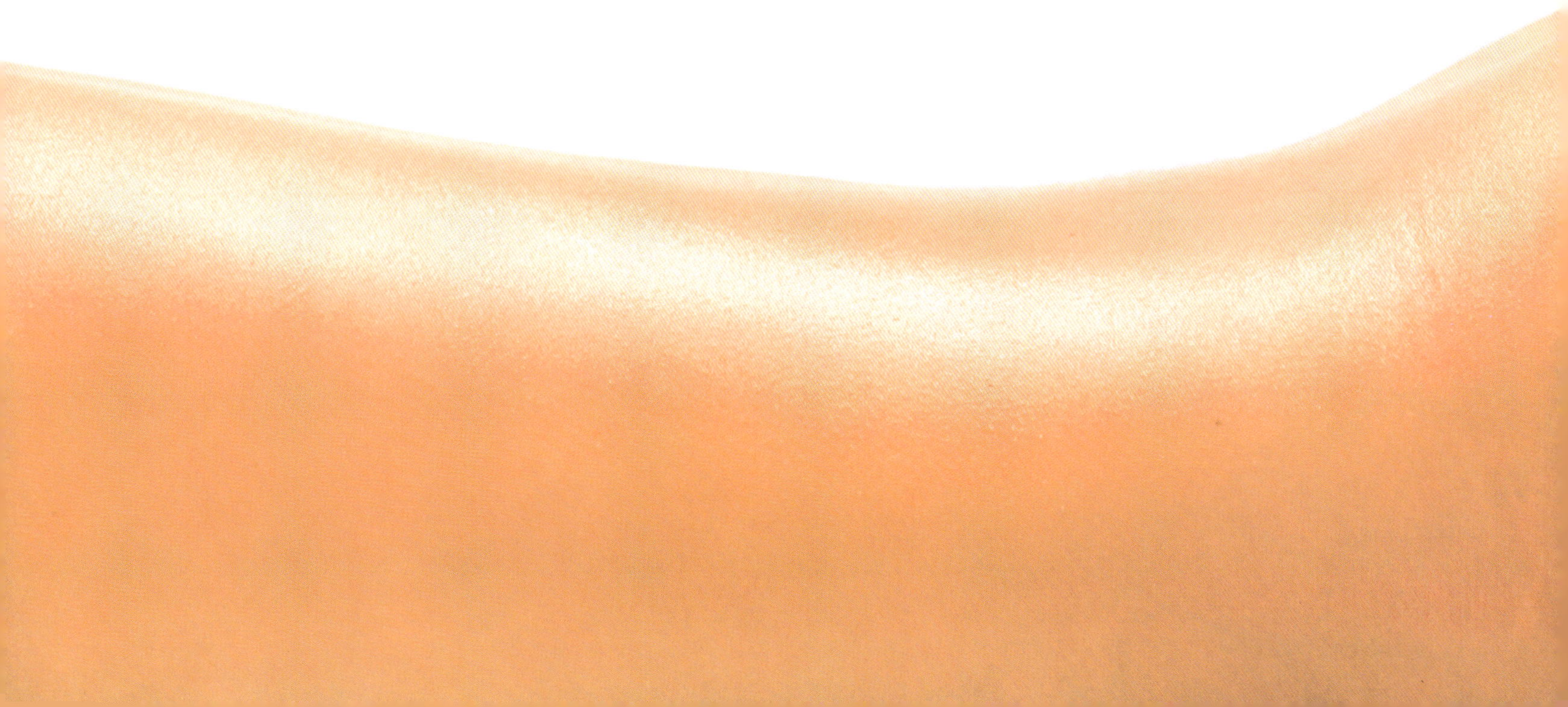

# essential oil safety: 1

Although essential oils are totally natural products, they come in a highly concentrated form and should always be used with respect and understanding. The safety guidelines discussed here are designed to help you gain the best therapeutic effects, with minimum risk, when giving aromatherapy massage.

The average bottled essential oil is approximately one hundred times stronger than the oil found in the original plant. As a result, essential oils are highly specialized natural substances that are also incredibly powerful – this is why they should only ever be used in very small amounts. There are several important safety guidelines that you need to understand when using essential oils; general points are covered here, and safety information regarding aromatherapy for special groups, such as the very young, older people and pregnant women, is discussed on pp.26–27. In addition, in Chapter 3, the Essential Oil Directory, you will see that each individual oil profile gives safety details regarding its use.

Aromatherapy massage should never be considered as a replacement for qualified medical advice or treatment. If you or someone you are treating have any specific physical or psychological symptoms, always ask a medical practitioner for advice. It may also help to consult a qualified aromatherapist for support and guidance in the safe use of essential oils.

## ESSENTIAL OIL SAFETY POINTS

You should always apply the following guidelines when using essential oils for aromatherapy massage.

### Always dilute essential oil

With one notable exception, (see the essential oil profile for lavender, p.93) you should never use essential oils neat on the skin. When giving an aromatherapy massage, you will use a blend made of specific amounts of essential oils diluted in a much greater amount of vegetable carrier oil. This is deliberate; the carrier oil performs the dual purpose of diluting the essential oil to a concentration that can be absorbed through the skin safely, in tiny amounts, and providing enough oil for you to massage a whole body.

Throughout chapters 2 and 3, I suggest many different blends for you to try, to suit the requirements of the person receiving the massage. Each one gives the exact number of drops to use of each oil. It is important that you follow the stated number of drops precisely. The blends given prescribe a dilution of 2.5 per cent; meaning that the essential oils account for just 2.5 per cent of the total amount of liquid. This is the safest dilution for general massage; in some specific cases, such as when massaging somone who is pregnant or has sensitive skin, the dilution will be reduced even further.

### Do not swallow essential oils

Essential oils could pose a toxicity risk if they come into immediate contact with the mucus lining of the mouth and digestive tract. The oils are highly concentrated and would be absorbed into the bloodstream far more quickly and in considerably higher amounts than when they are delivered through the skin during a massage. Essential oils should never be taken orally for any reason. If any oil is swallowed accidentally, seek medical attention immediately.

It is extremely important to keep all essential oils well out of the reach of infants and small children who are most at risk from accidental oral dosage.

### Be careful with sensitive or damaged skin

If your skin, or the skin of anyone on whom you are performing aromatherapy massage, is sensitive to perfumes or toiletry products, for example if it reddens or breaks out into rashes, add only half the stated number of drops of essential oils in any blend you use. For example, if a normal blend dilution is 4 drops of lavender and 6 drops of sweet orange in 4tsp (20ml) carrier oil, a sensitive skin blend would contain only 2 drops of lavender and 3 drops of sweet orange in the same amount (4tsp/20ml) of carrier oil. This guideline also applies if the skin you are treating ever suffers from skin-damaging problems, such as eczema or psoriasis.

The following essential oils should not be used on sensitive or damaged skin: may chang, tea tree, lemongrass, Scotch pine and ylang ylang. This is because they all contain potentially skin-sensitizing chemicals. If you have chosen a blend containing one of these oils, you need to replace the oil with a milder substitute, as well as making the blend at half the dilution.

### Avoid allergic reactions

One of the most important things you can do to avoid triggering allergic reactions to an essential oil is to ensure that oils are only ever used in blends, and never applied neat to the skin. If the person you want to massage has a tendency to allergic skin reactions, you should avoid the oils prohibited for sensitive skin (listed above) and, again, make any massage blends at half the number of stated drops.

If the person you are massaging experiences any kind of reaction while you are working on their skin, stop using your blend immediately. Wash it off straightaway with an unfragranced gentle soap and water, and apply a plain carrier such as grapeseed oil to the area – this should soothe any itching very quickly. If you are using blends at the dilutions given in this book, the likelihood of provoking an allergic reaction is extremely rare.

### Be careful in the sun

Essential oils from the citrus family – lemon, grapefruit, sweet orange and mandarin – contain a constituent called bergaptene which can cause skin sensitivity in ultra-violet light and lead to the formation of patches of irregular pigmentation. If you apply a massage blend containing any of these oils, advise the recipient to avoid exposing their skin to direct sunlight or a sunbed for 12 hours after application.

### Be careful with high blood pressure

If you are massaging a person who suffers from high blood pressure, do not use rosemary oil in your blend as it has a very stimulating effect on the circulation. Try replacing it with a more soothing oils, such as lavender or sandalwood.

### Be careful with epilepsy

Sufferers of epilepsy are normally well aware of their condition and manage it. They are susceptible to electrical disturbances in the brain, which can cause seizures or epileptic fits. The use of rosemary or yarrow essential oils can potentially increase the rate of epileptic seizures because of their highly stimulating effects on the brain; they should be avoided when treating people with epilepsy. However, research has also shown that using calming oils, such as ylang ylang or lavender, can help reduce seizure rates and induce a state of deep relaxation, and some epilepsy patients use aromatherapy to help manage their condition.

# essential oil safety: 2

In addition to the general safety guidelines discussed on the previous pages, here is some advice for giving massage with essential oils to certain groups – pregnant women, babies and young children, and older people – all of whom have special needs but who can also benefit greatly from the therapeutic effects of a treatment.

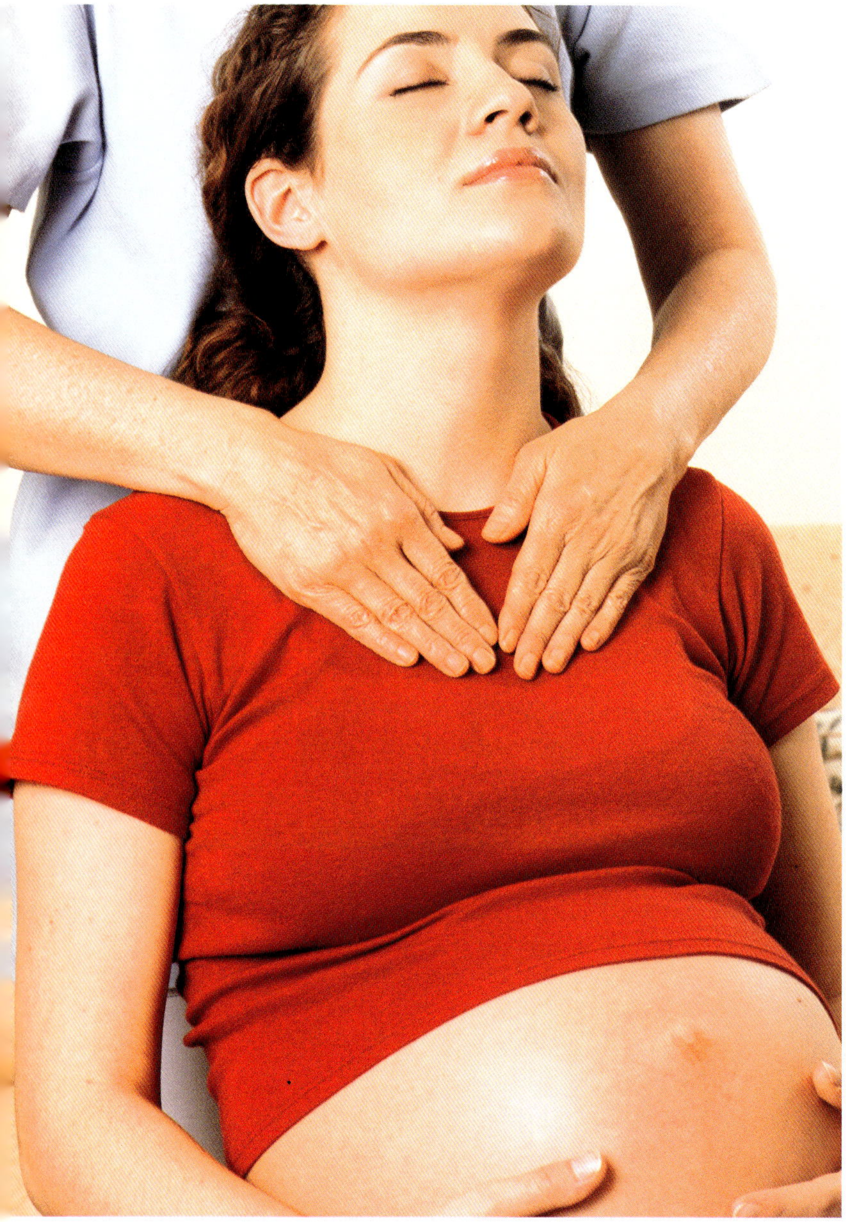

The blends quoted in this book are calculated to be mild on the skin yet effective in massage. However, sometimes they need to be diluted further, to ensure that the person receiving the massage is treated appropriately. Here are some circumstances when this applies.

**AROMATHERAPY IN PREGNANCY**

It is of utmost importance that you work safely when giving a massage to somebody who is pregnant. A relaxing massage, once or twice a week, is highly beneficial to an expectant mother, especially as she nears the end of her pregnancy and prepares for labour. Any treatment should be very gentle and should concentrate on smooth, flowing movements. Essential oils enhance a treatment – use those that are relaxing and soothing to body and mind, such as lavender or neroli. If you are unsure about any aspect of giving a massage to someone who is pregnant, ask a qualified aromatherapist for advice. Also make sure that the mother-to-be has consulted her midwife.

Any blends used on pregnant women must keep the same amount of carrier oil but contain only half the number of essential oil drops quoted in the formula. Essential oils must never be swallowed as internal absorption could be harmful to both mother and unborn baby. Use of certain oils is particularly beneficial during pregnancy, while others are considered too powerful and should be avoided. The most beneficial oils to use in pregnancy are: cardamom, Roman and German

| MASSAGE BLENDS FOR BABIES AND YOUNG CHILDREN | | |
|---|---|---|
| | BLENDS | BENEFITS |
| BABIES (6–18 months) | *1 drop essential oil in 4tsp (20ml) carrier oil (a dilution of 0.25%)* | |
| | **Either** Lavender 1 drop | soothes skin; calming; relaxing |
| | **or** Rose 1 drop | soothes skin; reduces soreness and nappy rash |
| | **or** Roman Chamomile 1 drop | soothes skin; reduces redness and sore skin |
| INFANTS (18 months to 4 years) | *4 drops essential oil in 4tsp (20ml) carrier oil (a dilution of 1%)* | |
| | **Either** Lavender 2 drops and Roman chamomile 2 drops | relaxing and calming |
| | **or** Sweet orange 2 drops and Rosewood 2 drops | soothing and uplifting |
| | **or** Rose 2 drops and Mandarin 2 drops | soothing and helps digestion |
| YOUNG CHILDREN (4 years to 12 years) | *8 drops essential oil in 4tsp (20ml) carrier oil (a dilution of 2%)* | |
| | **Either** Ginger 3 drops and Lavender 5 drops | warming and soothing; helps indigestion |
| | **or** Grapefruit 4 drops and Rosemary 4 drops | warming and fresh; helps aching muscles |
| | **or** Lavender 4 drops, Eucalyptus 2 drops and Cardamom 2 drops | helps as a chest rub for colds and flu |

chamomile, coriander seed, geranium, ginger, lavender, lemon, mandarin, neroli, patchouli, petitgrain, rose, rosewood, sweet orange and sandalwood. Essential oils to avoid when pregnant are: fennel, rosemary, yarrow, juniper berry, myrhh, angelica, basil and Spanish sage.

## AROMATHERAPY FOR BABIES AND CHILDREN

The blends quoted in chapters 2 and 3 are safe dilutions for adults and children over the age of 12. However, for younger children and babies the oil in blends needs to be at a much lower dilution. This is because young skin is much finer than adult skin, and absorbs more of the essential oils, so smaller amounts are needed.

Baby massage is popular in many cultures; it promotes the parent–child bond and gives the baby a sense of security and well-being. Massage can also help babies to gain weight and research suggests it boosts their immune systems too. Newborns are best massaged with a good-quality, plain carrier oil such as sweet almond, or a specialist carrier oil such as kukui nut (see pp.30–31). Once a child is six months old, you can use a massage blend (see table, above).

## AROMATHERAPY FOR OLDER PEOPLE

Aromatherapy massage can also be highly effective for older people. During massage we experience caring touch – something older people often lack – and it can lift our mood. The use of essential oils adds a pleasant and often evocative element to treatment. In fact, essential oils are now sometimes used in the treatment of patients with memory problems because their fragrance can help to stimulate the memory.

Most massage for older people concentrates on areas that are easily accessible, such as the hands, feet, face, or neck and shoulders, as the elderly often find a full body massage too daunting. When using blends on older people it is important to halve the number of drops while keeping the same amount of carrier oil, as the skin tends to thin with age. Also bear in mind the cautions regarding high blood pressure and epilepsy (see p.25). Hand massage is particularly good because the scent of the essential oils lingers there and can be enjoyed afterward. The combination of touch and smell can encourage and enhance communication between carers and older people.

# buying and storing essential oils

Once you begin to collect essential oils you need to know how long to keep them and how to store them properly. The oils are natural substances and will degrade over time, particularly if they are over-exposed to air, light or heat. Follow the advice given here and enjoy building and taking care of your essential oil collection.

It is important to buy and use oils as fresh as possible; as they begin to degrade, their composition changes and this could cause skin sensitivity. Following a few simple rules will help you to get the most from your oils.

### CHOOSING A SUPPLIER

Essential oils are now readily available from good chemists, drugstores, and health food shops; these are the best retail sources to choose because they are likely to have a good turnover of stock and, therefore, the freshest oils. Buying from trade suppliers is another option; many do mail order, but often they require you to have an aromatherapy qualification before they will sell to you. Good suppliers should be able to tell you how fresh their oils are and how often they replace them, and be able to answer any basic questions you may have. If you are given vague replies consider going elsewhere; it is better to buy from an informed source.

### BOTTLE DESIGN

Most oils come in small glass bottles with a 2tsp (10ml) capacity. Always buy essential oils in dark glass bottles – preferably dark brown or dark blue, because these colours help to protect the contents from ultra-violet (UV) light, which causes the oil to degrade. Avoid buying oils in clear glass bottles as these spoil quickly.

The bottle should have a screw top which fits tightly and also, importantly, a special insert in the neck. This is called a "dropper insert" and it enables the release of a slow and steady flow of drops when you tip up the bottle, so you can count the drops accurately. The dropper insert also helps protect against accidental swallowing – should it happen, the amounts would be tiny. Never buy essential oils sold in open-necked bottles for this reason.

### KEEPING YOUR ESSENTIAL OILS

To maximize the shelf life of your essential oils, you need to minimize their contact with air, heat and UV light. Air, or more specifically oxygen, reacts with the contents of essential oils and causes them to degrade over time. It is better to buy small bottles of oils and use them up regularly because there is very little air space in the bottles, even as the contents go down. Bottles should also be kept tightly closed when oils are in storage, and when you open the bottle to make a blend make sure you replace the lid as soon as possible.

Heat can speed up the degradation of essential oils considerably, so keep them as cool as possible. The best place to store them is in the refrigerator; doing so will double their shelf life. Finally, avoid UV light, as this also quickly degrades essential oils. This is why you should buy and store oils in dark glass bottles, and keep them out of direct light. If you don't keep your oils in the refrigerator, make sure they are in a cool, dark place.

The shelf life of an essential oil starts the day you open a fresh bottle; write this date on the lid or the label so you can see at a glance how old your oil is. Most essential oils have a shelf life of two years from opening if kept in the refrigerator, and a year from opening if kept in a cool, dark place (50–59°F/10–15°C). The exceptions to this are the citrus oils (orange, lemon, mandarin and grapefruit) and tea tree oil, which are affected by oxygen and light to a higher degree. These oils have a shelf life of one year from opening if kept in the refrigerator, and six months from opening if kept in a cool, dark place.

## IDENTIFYING AND DISPOSING OF OLD OILS

As well as the age of an essential oil, other factors may show that it has degraded. If there is a sudden change in aroma, with sour or rancid notes, or a cloudiness in the bottle, or a greatly diminished odour the oil should be discarded. Oils can be safely disposed of into the drainage system, and empty bottles rinsed and included in glass recycling. Do not be tempted to keep oils beyond their shelf life; it is much better to buy in fresh supplies.

## TRAVELLING WITH ESSENTIAL OILS

I never leave home without a basic kit of essential oils – lavender (for relaxation, sleep and headaches), tea tree (general antiseptic) and peppermint (for travel nausea, headaches or stomach problems). If I am going abroad, I usually take some more oils such as may chang and patchouli (insect repellents), and lemon or orange (good for room fragrancing). This kit is carried in a small airtight box which I take in my hand luggage. However, when travelling essential oils may be subject to changes in temperature, so I allow them only a short shelf life of half the normal amount of time, and I check them regularly for any signs of oxidization.

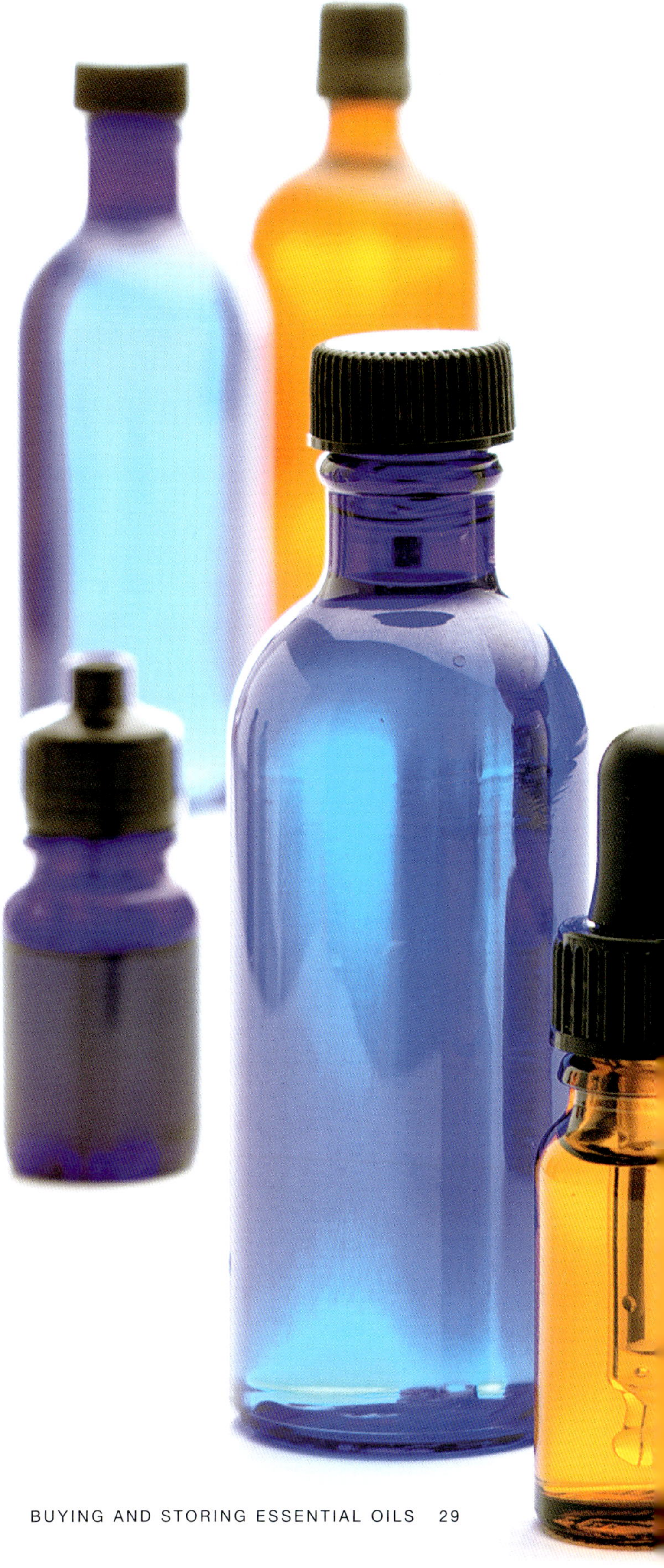

# making blends

The art of aromatherapy lies in making a balanced blend of essential oils in a suitable carrier oil, ready for you to apply to the skin using massage. This is an exciting and creative process which can achieve amazing results. Here you will find instructions on how to make a blend as well as information about carrier oils.

When you mix essential oils in a vegetable oil carrier, the molecules of the fragrances form new molecular chains and create a new aroma. There are countless possible combinations, making this is a highly creative aspect of aromatherapy. You should balance the fragrance of the blend so that no oils predominate, and choose a suitable carrier so that the skin is nourished and supple but not sticky at the end of the treatment. In chapters 2 and 3 you will find many choices of blends, which you can use to create wonderful massage treatments.

Measure out the carrier oil first, as this is the fatty medium which is needed to combine the essential oils into a new fragrance. Once you have made the mixture, it is important to shake it; this agitation improves the blending process, and has been called "the dance of the molecules". A 4tsp (20ml) blend should give you enough mixture to perform a substantial massage treatment, such as on the back, neck and shoulders, and for most people it will be enough to massage the whole body minus the face. If the recipient is very large or has a lot of body hair, you may need to double the quantity of carrier oil to 8tsp (40ml), and double the number of drops of each essential oil used in the formula too.

In practice it is preferable to make up a fresh blend each time you work. Using small amounts of carrier and fresh essential oils helps to minimize any potential skin reactions. Aromatherapy blends will keep for up to four weeks after they are made, in a cool, dark place, but you will probably find that you want to vary the essential oils you use and not stick with the same formula. The more

### HOW TO MAKE AN AROMATHERAPY BLEND

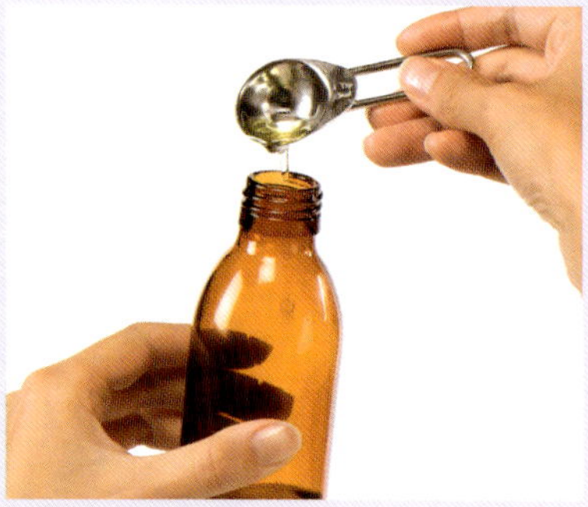

**STEP 1:** Carefully measure 4tsp (20ml) of your chosen carrier oil into a clean 10-tsp (50-ml) dark glass bottle.

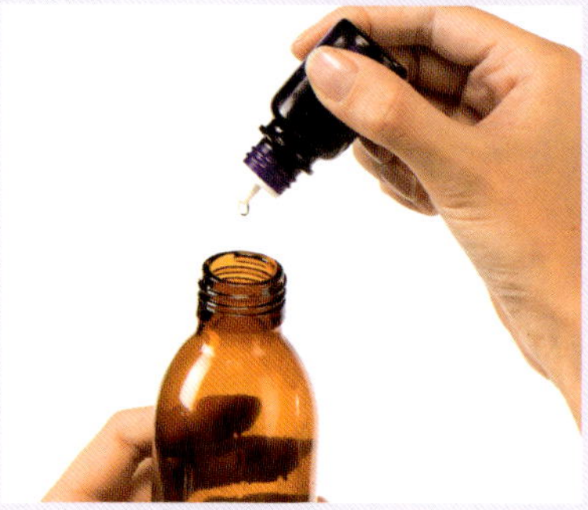

**STEP 2:** Add the correct number of drops of each essential oil from your chosen blend, counting them with care.

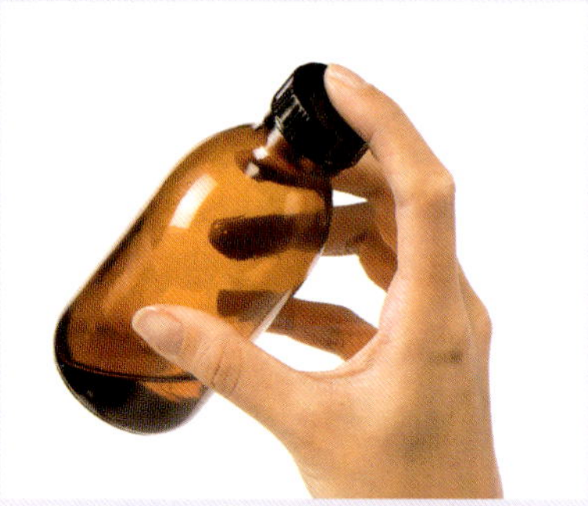

**STEP 3:** Screw the lid on the bottle tightly and give the mixture a vigorous shake. It is now ready to use.

## SELECTING CARRIER OILS

| BASIC CARRIERS | SPECIALIST CARRIERS |
|---|---|
| **Sweet Almond** (*Prunus amygdalus* var. *dulcis*)<br>A good, all-round, pale yellow carrier with high levels of minerals as well as the fatty oleic and linoleic acids, which are both excellent skin and hair conditioners. This is an excellent massage carrier for skins with tendency to dryness. | **Camellia** (*Camellia sasanqua*)<br>Made from Japanese camellia flowers, this lovely carrier is used extensively in the East for skin, hair and nail care; it keeps all three strong, supple and well-nourished. It is light to work with in massage and leaves a silky finish. |
| **Jojoba** (*Simmondsia chinensis*)<br>Golden yellow in colour, jojoba is an excellent all-round skin conditioner taken from the beans of the jojoba bush. It has a different composition to most carrier oils – it is actually a liquid wax. It is similar to the skin's own oil, sebum, and works on any skin type to improve texture and hydration. It can be used for face or body massage. | **Kukui Nut** (*Aleurites moluccana*)<br>The kukui tree is the Hawaiian national tree, and the oil from the nuts is used extensively in Hawaii for massage for all age groups – even newborn babies, who are anointed with it just after birth. This carrier oil helps the skin to regenerate when there is eczema or psoriasis present – both of these conditions damage the upper skin layers. |
| **Grapeseed** (*Vitis vinifera*)<br>This is a much lighter pale green carrier and is good for skins that are already well-hydrated, such as olive complexions, or skins with a tendency to oiliness. It leaves little residue and is easy to work with, especially in body massage. | **Macadamia Nut** (*Macadamia integrifolia* and *M. tetraphylla*)<br>This rich carrier from Australia is also excellent for very young or very old skins which are thinner, more delicate and therefore more vulnerable. You can use it for body massage and it is very helpful for extremely dry skin. |
| **Apricot Kernel** (*Prunus armeniaca*)<br>This light-textured, almost colourless carrier is particularly good for facial massage because it does not clog the pores but leaves the skin silky and supple. It contains oleic and linoleic fatty acids in high amounts, which supply excellent nourishment to the skin. | **Avocado** (*Persea americana*)<br>This deep green carrier made from avocado pulp has a very thick consistency (you can combine it with a lighter carrier if you wish) and contains skin-nourishing vitamins A and D, potassium and lecithin. Avocado oil is particularly recommended for extremely dry skin. |

blends you make, the more practice you get and the more confident you will become in using essential oils.

Choose wide-necked bottles for your blends, as these are easier to wash out after treatments. Use very hot water and a good detergent to get all the old blend out of the bottle, then thoroughly rinse and leave to dry.

### CARRIER OILS

These are the golden tools of aromatherapy massage which supply nourishment and care to the skin. They are all vegetable oils, extracted from seeds and nuts full of nutrients that are vital to healthy skin. Petroleum products such as Vaseline, or mineral oils such as baby oil are not used in aromatherapy as they are barriers, which prevent the skin from breathing, and are slippery, making massage more difficult. In aromatherapy massage the carrier oil is very important because it not only delivers the blend to the skin but also cares for the skin layers, improving cell renewal and enhancing the outer texture.

When buying carrier oils for aromatherapy, you need top-quality vegetable oils, which are as unrefined as possible. Many are available at organic standard and "cold pressed", which means they are processed at cool temperatures, preserving vitamin content. These are available from health-food shops or drugstores. Trade suppliers also sell quality carrier oils. These oils have a shelf life of between six and nine months, and should be kept out of direct sunlight in a cool place.

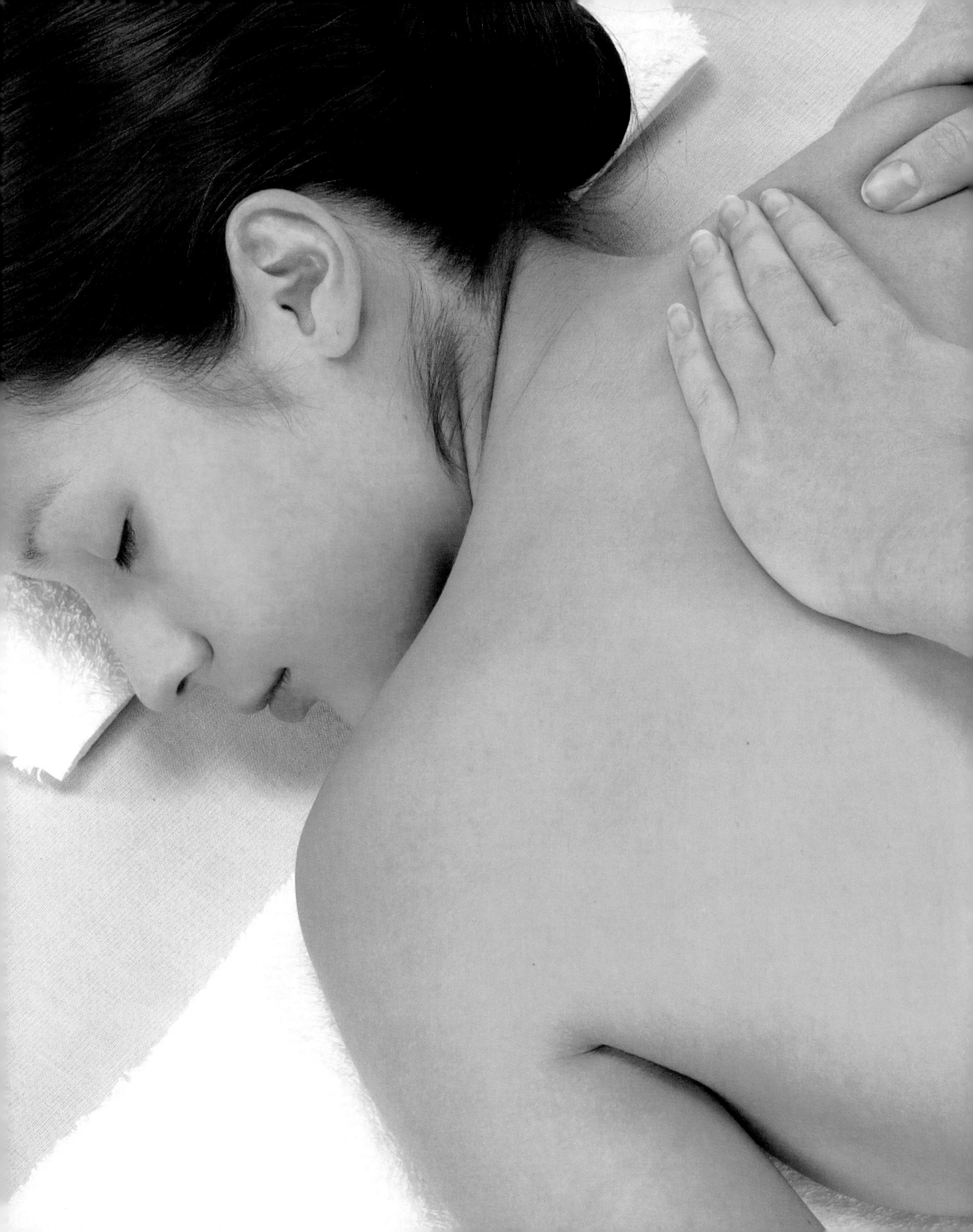

CHAPTER TWO

# aromatherapy massage

*Massage is the most effective way of giving aromatherapy to another person. It is a form of caring touch that is an art form in itself, but when combined with an aromatic essential oil blend, the whole experience takes the recipient to another level of relaxation and well-being.*

In this chapter we learn about massage as a healing tool, take a look at its historical background and discover some of the specific benefits that using essential oils may bring to a treatment. I advise you on how to approach the giving of massage, and offer practical advice on setting up your massage space. There are detailed descriptions of all the basic massage strokes, and step-by-step routines suggested for the different parts of the body, each with a selection of essential oil blends for you to try. The routines, which include some for self-massage, are all designed to be simple to apply so you can learn them easily. You may feel that your first attempts are unsure, but the more you practise giving caring touch, the more your confidence will grow. As you learn this new skill and share it with the people around you, above all enjoy it!

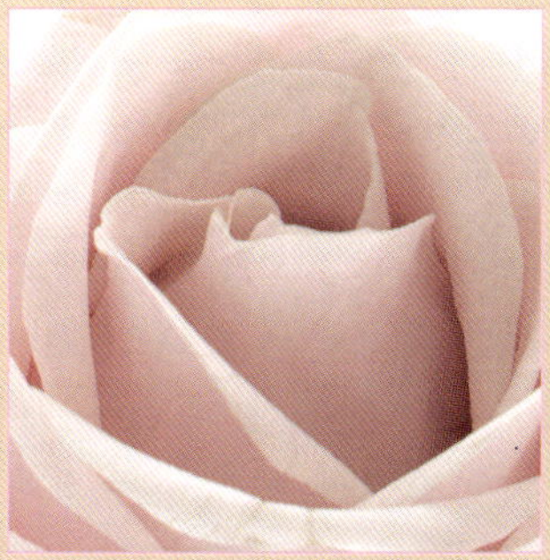

# what is massage?

In many ways massage is a continuation of the sense of touch, but is a more precise and deliberate way of applying it. Since earliest times, humans have employed this kind of deliberate touch in various forms always with the aim of helping the recipient and improving their physical and mental well-being.

We all know how instinctive it is to rub an area which hurts, or to squeeze a tense muscle to ease pain. We might also use a pat of the hand or gentle pressure to reassure someone who is in distress. We begin to learn about touch from the moment we are born and held as tiny infants in the arms of our parents. The more caring touch we receive as babies, the better we grow and the stronger our immune system becomes. This has been proven many times, one famous example being a study from early 20th-century New York where, in a large orphanage, scientists observed that babies who were held a lot by the nurses (probably because of their appearance and their ability to hold good eye contact with the nurses) gained more weight and were far healthier than those who were not held as much.

**MASSAGE IN THE PAST**

Massage is as old as humankind; evidence from prehistoric times points to the use of herbs, spices and other ingredients, which were rubbed on the body for healing, often by a medicine man or woman. This practice still survives in some places, for example among the peoples of the Amazon where ointments and pastes made of herbs and fat are rubbed onto the body.

Ancient Egyptian tomb paintings show different types of massage to the face, the feet and the torso, and it is known that the pharaohs and members of the high nobility were massaged daily. The Ancient Greeks were also aware of the value of massage as a healing tool. Hippocrates (c. 460–377 BCE), known as the father of modern medicine, advocated massage as a way of improving stiff muscles and aching joints; he specifically advised the use of rubbing or friction to increase heat to the area. Galen, a Roman physician of the 2nd century CE, wrote many books on the subject of massage and advised it for gladiators before and after combat.

In India the Ayurvedic system of medicine, which is over 2,000 years old, advocated massage of the body, scalp and hair using aromatic oils every morning after bathing. Massage was also appreciated in the ancient Arab culture: in the 10th century the famous physician and scholar Abu-Ibn-Sina (Avicenna) wrote of the benefits of massage, bathing and exercise to improve health.

**MASSAGE TODAY**

For centuries many cultures have used touch and massage to help and heal humankind from babyhood, and continue to do so to this day. Many African mothers carry their infants wrapped on their backs, so their movements lull the child to sleep as it feels and smells the presence of its mother. In Hawaii newborn babies are immediately massaged with kukui nut oil, which has special moisturizing and hydrating properties, helping the baby's skin to adapt to the hot humid environment. In many cultures massage is given daily to all members of the family. It is a simple and instinctive exchange.

In some northern European countries there tends to be more reserve when it comes to massage and touch,

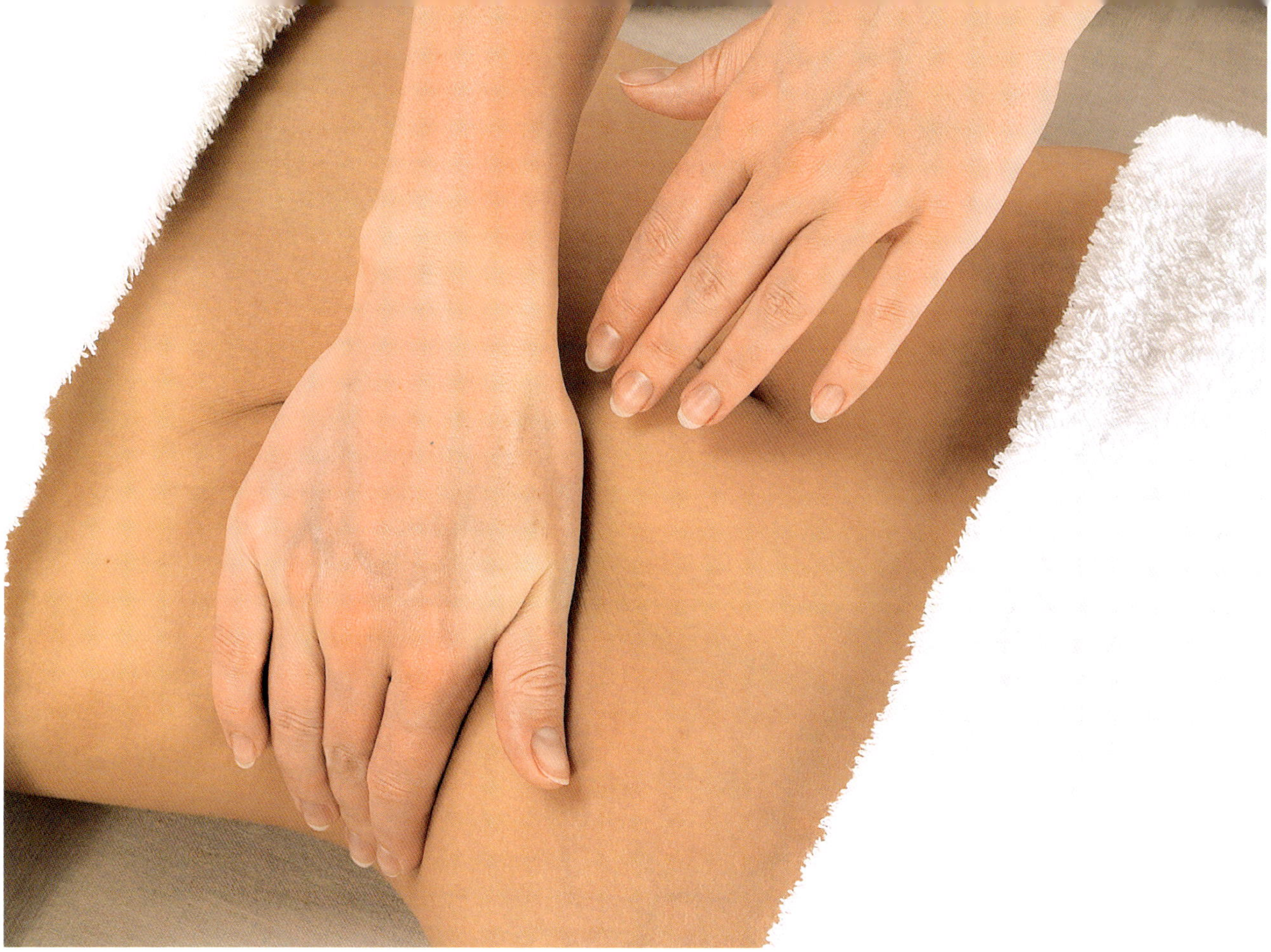

and this has become exaggerated to the point where there is almost a fear of it. This is because the notion of touch and sexual contact has become confused. Massage has gained a reputation as having sexual connotations, and this interferes with its acceptance as a safe and non-sexual way of improving well-being. Of course touch is involved in sex, but it is in a totally different context. Simple caring touch is what massage is all about, and what we are here to learn. If you feel and experience gentle, confident and respectful touch, you will soon realize its value and beneficial effects.

## GIVING MASSAGE

When you give massage to someone else it can be just as powerful an experience as receiving it. As the giver, a person is trusting you to treat them with care. In one Ancient Egyptian wall painting, a patient is saying to a practitioner "Please do not hurt me", and the response from the therapist is "I shall act so I praise you". This is crucial to understanding the massage exchange; giving massage is an act of care, with the purposeful intention to give a wonderful and supportive experience. If you do this, you are certainly praising the recipient, as well as giving them a gift of improved well-being.

You can, of course, give massage to yourself – at least to a degree. As a therapist I have taught self-massage to many clients over the years, and it has been another way to help them re-learn the value of caring touch. For example, a gentle clockwise self-massage of the abdomen, with a pain-soothing aromatherapy blend, followed by the application of a hot water bottle is a highly effective and soothing treatment for menstrual pain. Foot treatments such as a foot soak, scrub and a self-given foot massage are a lovely treat at the end of a long, hard day. And while you are not able to massage your own back, you can work on your shoulders to relieve aches and pains and achieve good results. Self-treatment is not as effective as receiving a massage from someone else, but it is still beneficial. You will find some routines to try later in this chapter (see pp.78–85).

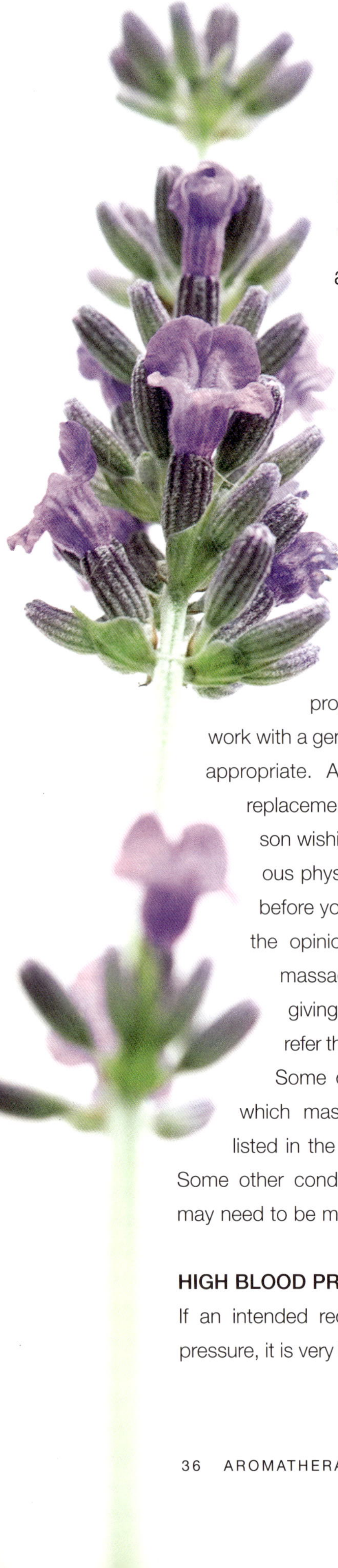

# massage safety

If you are going to give someone massage you must do it in a safe way. You need to apply massage techniques with sensitivity and an awareness of the recipient's particular needs. There are some circumstances in which massage definitely should not be used, especially if you are a beginner. Take note of the advice below before you begin.

Trained massage therapists may work in special circumstances to a degree, because they have studied anatomy and physiology and know how to apply more complex techniques. If you are a beginner, be aware that areas on which you plan to work must be warmed up properly before you begin. Always start work with a gentle pressure, increasing this slowly as appropriate. And remember, massage is not a replacement for medical treatment – if the person wishing to receive massage has any obvious physical symptoms, seek medical advice before you begin. It may also be helpful to ask the opinion of a qualified aromatherapist or massage therapist. If you are unsure about giving a massage, refrain from working and refer the person concerned to a professional.

Some of the most common conditions for which massage may not be appropriate are listed in the table of contraindications, opposite. Some other conditions for which massage treatment may need to be modified are discussed below.

## HIGH BLOOD PRESSURE

If an intended recipient has a history of high blood pressure, it is very important to work with smooth gentle movements only; fast, vigorous massage and deep pressure can increase the circulation and, therefore, the burden on the heart. However, gentle, flowing massage can actually lower blood pressure.

## HEART DISEASE AND STROKE

A person with a known and identified heart condition, such as angina or coronary heart disease, or a history of strokes, requires only gentle, flowing massage and no vigorous or deep movements, so as to avoid overburdening the circulation and heart. Gentle treatment will have a beneficial effect.

## PREGNANCY

Massage is highly beneficial during pregnancy. It must be smooth, flowing and carefully applied, avoiding any deep pressures or more stimulating movements such as cupping. It should be a pleasant and soothing experience for the recipient. If you are unsure about how to work, seek the advice of a professional massage therapist or aromatherapist. It is also important for the mother-to-be to consult her midwife about receiving massage. See also Essential Oil Safety: 2, page 26.

## CANCER

A great deal of professional support through the medium of massage is now available to cancer patients, and caring touch has extremely beneficial emotional

| MASSAGE CONTRAINDICATIONS | | |
|---|---|---|
| CONDITION | SYMPTOMS | ADVICE |
| Fever | A high temperature, which means that the body is coping with some kind of infection. | Massage should not be used as it would further stress the system. |
| Headache/Migraine | For headaches, a dull pain is often felt in the forehead or behind the eyes. For migraines the pain is much more severe, possibly with nausea, light disturbances and pain up the back of the head or over one eye. | In both cases, massage is not advised as its stimulating effects can make the conditions worse, particularly in the case of migraines. Rest and quiet are recommended. |
| Varicose veins | These are damaged veins, usually in the lower legs, with a raised or twisted appearance. The skin covering them tends to be thin. | No pressure should ever be applied to a damaged vein. It is possible, however, to apply gentle massage above and below an affected area, to improve general circulation. |
| Osteoporosis | This condition, mostly affecting post-menopausal women, causes the bones to become brittle. The vertebrae in the neck are particularly vulnerable. | Deep massage or pressure is not appropriate, but gentle massage can ease muscular tension. |
| Acute infectious conditions | This might be a viral episode such as influenza or a head cold, where the body is weak because it is fighting infection. | Massage is not used in these circumstances as it places additional stress on the system. |
| Inflammation | A red or swollen area on the body. Pay particular attention if it occurs around any joints, as this may indicate rheumatoid arthritis. | Massage of an inflamed area can exacerbate the problem and cause pain, so it should not be used. |
| Oedema | A pooling of fluid, often seen in the lower legs as puffiness or swelling. An example of its occurence might be after a long flight in an aircraft. | Specialist massage techniques are used by professionals to help oedema, but non-professionals are advised not to work as such a condition can have deeper medical implications. |
| Physical injury | Any physical trauma, such as bruising, sports' injury, ligament damage or severely torn muscles. | Only professional massage treatment should be given for these conditions. |

effects on sufferers. However, because of the complex nature of cancer and the medical treatments given for the condition, it is advisable for any sufferers to seek professional massage treatment.

Do not be put off from giving massage by these guidelines. Remember that if you are working safely, your treatment can only be beneficial. Safety information is given to build your confidence in what you are able to do. It can be helpful to make a list of potential problem areas, and to run through it with the person seeking treatment before you start working; if any of the conditions apply, you can then decide if it is appropriate for you to work at this time. Very often common sense will tell you whether or not it is advisable to proceed – you will find that in the vast majority of cases it is.

# the effects of massage

No other treatment makes you more aware of the power and complexity of the sense of touch than massage. As well as feeling the restorative physical effects, you will also quickly notice its beneficial effect on your mind and your mental state. To find out why, we need to take an in-depth look at an incredible organ – the skin.

The skin is not just a semi-waterproof covering. As we have already seen, it has three layers: the top layer (the epidermis) with overlapping cells; the middle layer (the dermis) with nourishing blood vessels; and the lower layer, the subcutaneous fat. The nerve endings, which are housed in the epidermis, are concerned with the sense of touch. In particular areas, such as the pads under the fingertips, there are clusters of nerves through which we perceive exquisitely subtle tactile impressions. Every hair follicle also has associated nerve endings – which is why it hurts when someone pulls your hair.

About one square inch (6.5cm$^2$) of skin contains more than 20 million cells, roughly 1200 sweat glands, at least 300 nerve endings and around 20ft (6m) of blood vessels. There are about 50 nerve receptors, which gather nerve impulses, to roughly every 1½in$^2$ (10cm$^2$) of skin, and a human body is estimated to have more than 600,000 receptors in total. These combine into sensory nerve fibres, of which approximately half a million enter the spine and the spinal cord to connect to the brain.

Inside the brain itself, the areas that receive and interpret the sense of touch are more extensive than those linked to the other senses, showing how very important touch has become in human evolution. The lips, tongue, finger pads and the upper and lower surfaces of the feet and hands are connected to particularly large areas of the brain – this is because they are the main parts of our bodies that come into direct contact with our environment. It also explains why the hands, the major tools for giving massage, are so important to both the recipient, who feels their touch, and to the giver, who feels and interprets information about the recipient through them. This is how massage becomes a form of communication.

There are also different types of skin receptors just under the skin's surface. Some are called mechanical receptors, because they simply convey an idea of pressure; they can also be linked to the sense of pain if pressure becomes too hard. Some are temperature receptors, which immediately react to heat or cold. Another group are called pain receptors. These respond like a reflex to injury, and are connected to motor nerves which make us jump or move away from anything threatening; they are also linked to feelings of anxiety or threat. These types of receptors show how sensitive the skin is, and how important it is that massage is given as caring touch.

Massage has known beneficial effects on the following parts of the body.

**MUSCLE TISSUE**

Massage increases the blood-flow through muscles, by literally "washing" them through with fresh blood. This brings the muscles nutrients to aid cellular renewal, as well as removing the toxins that cause fibres to stiffen and create tight or painful areas. Smooth, flowing movements achieve this effect, as well as more stimulating percussive movements, which increase local circulation in the blood vessels immediately under the skin.

### THE CIRCULATORY SYSTEM

Massage improves the blood's circulation generally, particularly when the massage is given over the whole body. Movements such as stroking, wringing and kneading help to release the soft tissue, allowing the blood to circulate more freely through it. This is very beneficial because it lets the body move better, alleviates stiffness and improves physical performance and stamina.

### THE LYMPHATIC SYSTEM

The body system known as the lymphatic system is intricately linked to the circulation. Through lymphatic vessels all over the body, a fluid called lymph aids the removal of toxins. Specialist massage techniques, such as lymphatic drainage, encourage the lymph to circulate through the body more efficiently; leg massage also has this effect. You can help the lymphatic system by taking regular exercise, such as walking. Sitting around can encourage lymphatic fluid to stagnate and pool, particularly in the legs.

### MOOD AND FEELINGS

Touch is interpreted in the cerebral cortex area of the brain, which also triggers our emotions. This area also controls our response to stress. In addition, the limbic system, which governs the sense of smell resides deep within the brain. The sensation of touch transmitted through the sensory nerves, and the sense of smell through the olfactory nerves, come together to trigger memories, feelings and emotions, and enhance relaxation. This is the magic of aromatherapy massage.

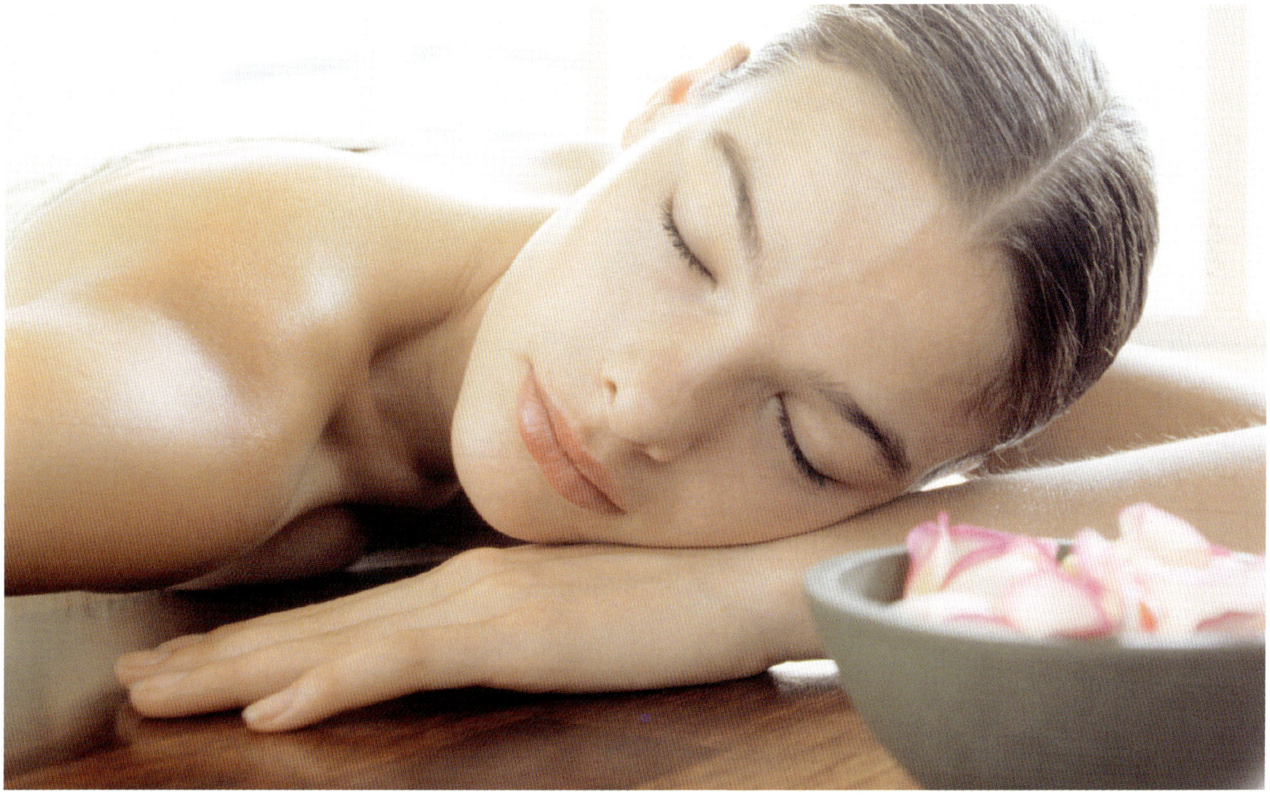

# basic massage strokes: 1

Massage means learning to use your hands in different ways. There are some classic strokes that are used regularly in many routines; it is helpful to learn how to do these individually before you start putting them together into treatment routines.

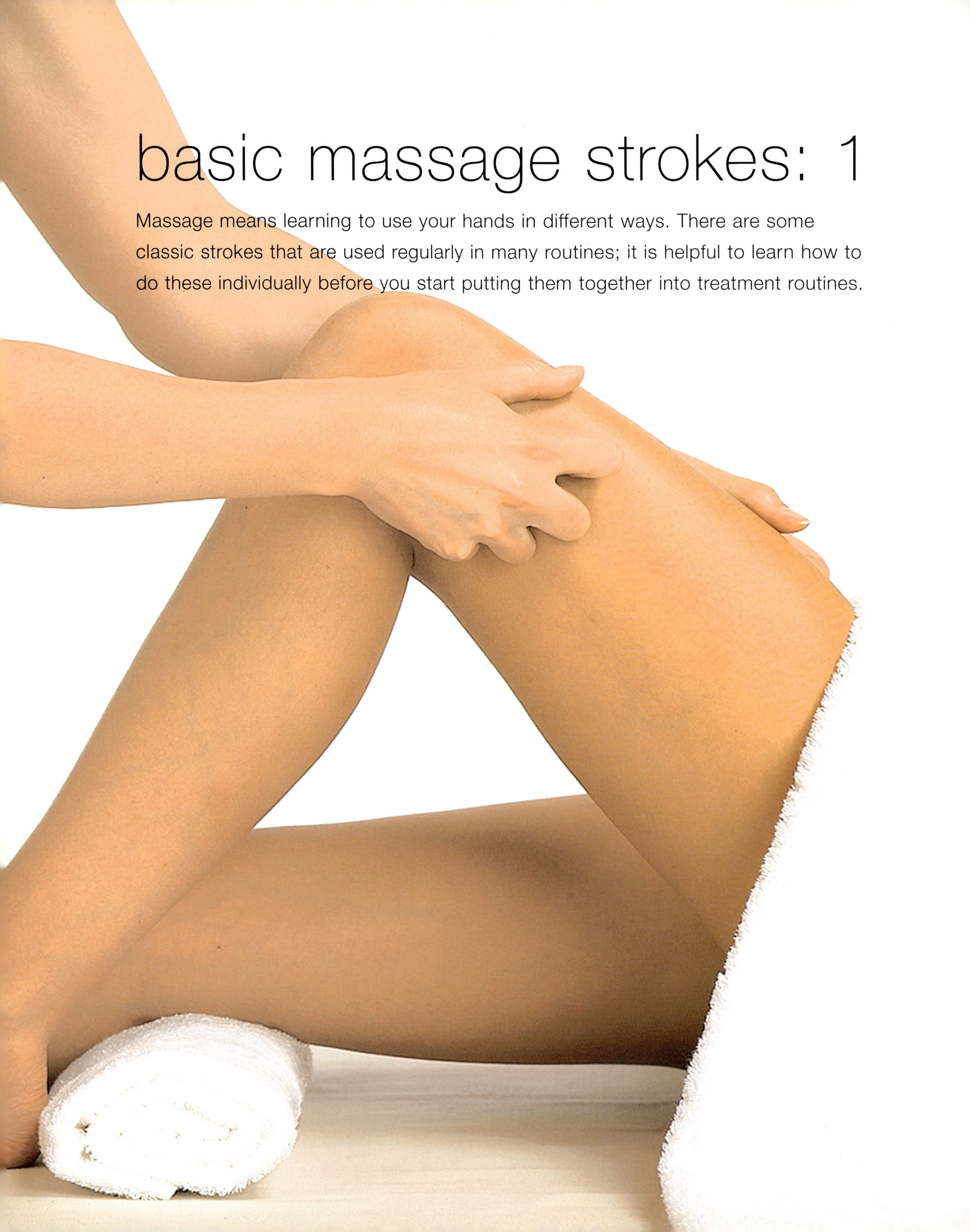

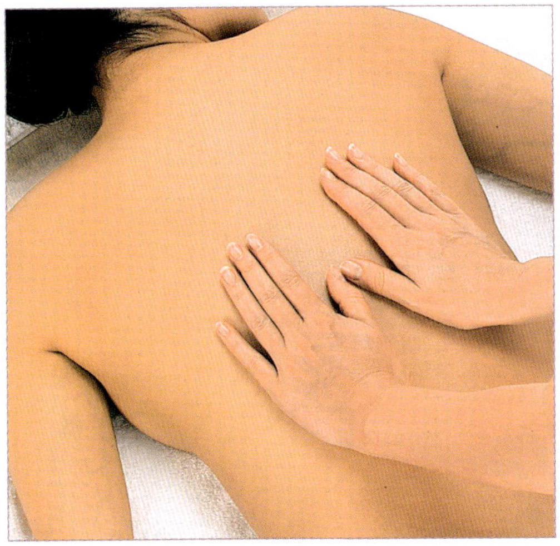

## EFFLEURAGE

This simply means "stroking". It is the most basic massage movement, and uses the whole of the palm of the hand. Effleurage really warms up the skin, easing away aches and pains. If you apply it quickly and vigorously, it feels more stimulating to receive; if you work more slowly, it feels very relaxing. You can use both hands together or just one hand on a small area.

*To try effleurage, work on someone's back. Stroke up either side of the spine toward the shoulders, down the sides of the back and up again. Repeat these movements several times.*

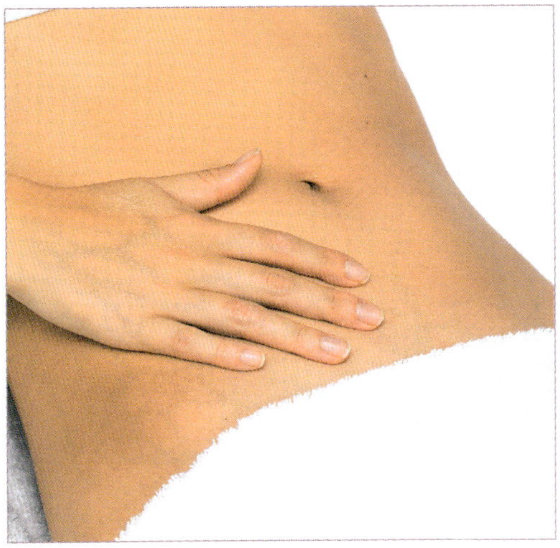

## CIRCLE STROKING

This is a different type of effleurage, where the movement is a definite circular motion across the skin. You can use just one hand or both hands if you wish. Circle stroking is particularly effective when applied to the abdomen to relieve menstrual cramps or indigestion, and has a warming effect.

*Try circle stroking on yourself. Place your right hand near your right hip, stroke up toward your ribs, over your stomach, down to your left hip and back across to where you started. Repeat this several times. Work in a clockwise direction as this is the correct direction to help your large intestine do its work of elimination.*

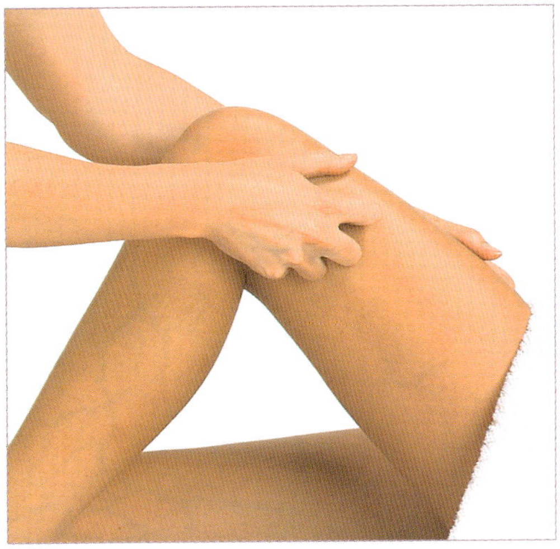

## KNUCKLING

Here is a more stimulating stroke, which is given with a slightly clenched fist, using your knuckles to create pressure. It should feel stronger as a movement, but the aim is not to cause pain. You need a little oil to lubricate the skin when you practise this stroke.

*Try it on another person, on the outer thigh. First apply a little carrier oil to the thigh, then slightly clench your fist. Using your knuckles, make lots of small circular movements up and down over the area. This is a good stroke to use to break down toxins in muscle fibres, aiding their elimination.*

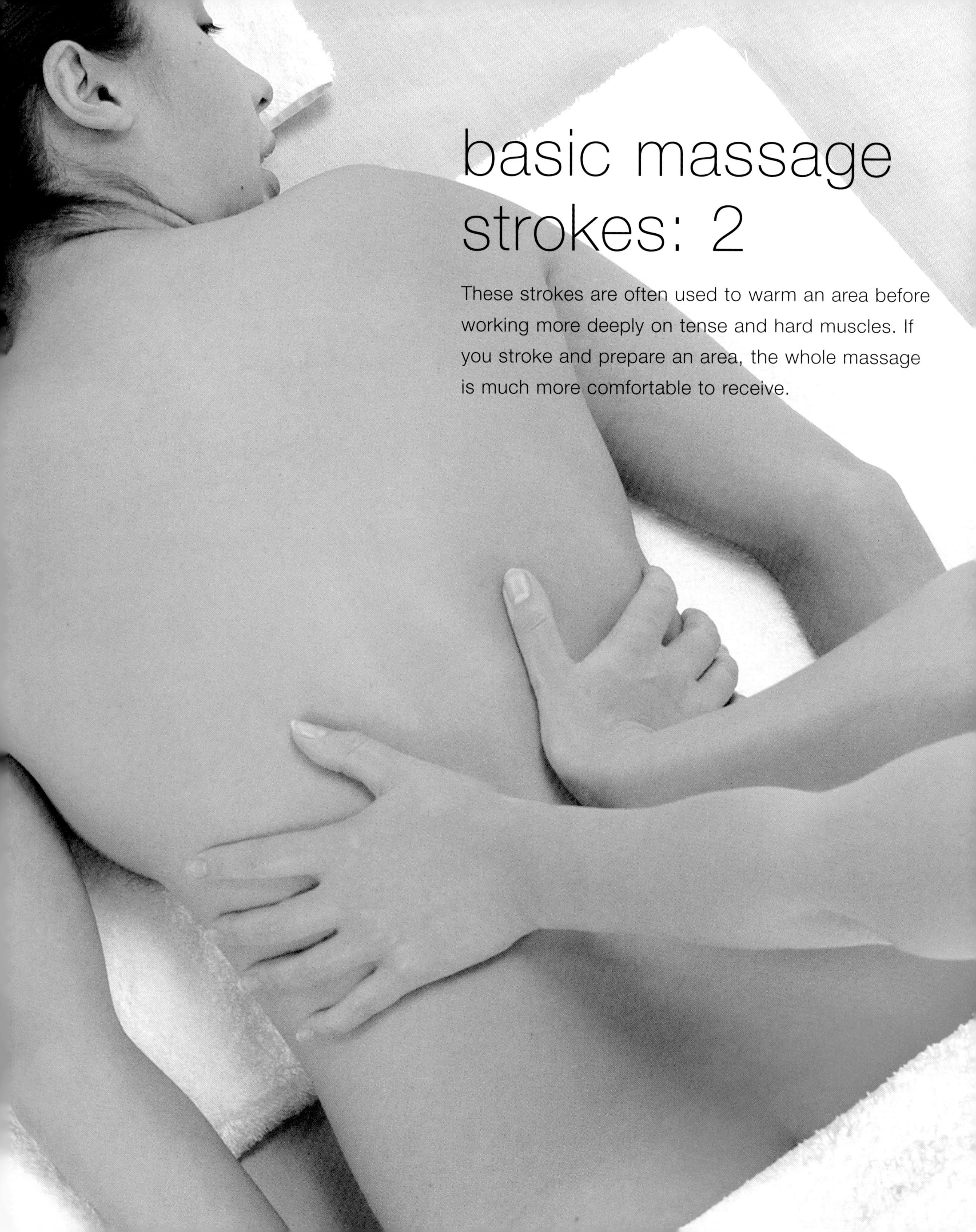

# basic massage strokes: 2

These strokes are often used to warm an area before working more deeply on tense and hard muscles. If you stroke and prepare an area, the whole massage is much more comfortable to receive.

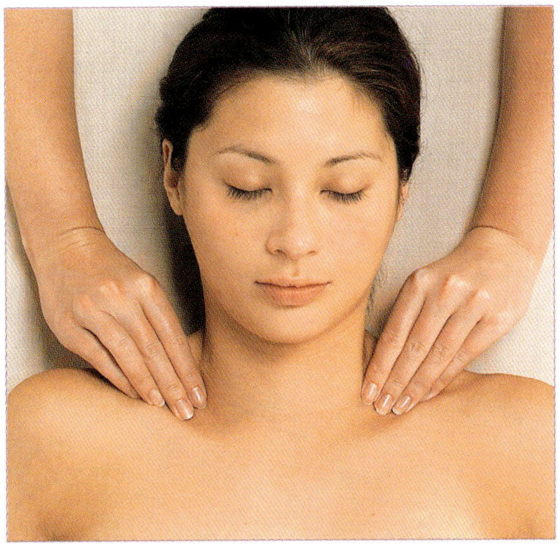

### SINGLE-HANDED KNEADING

This stroke is especially good for a very muscular area such as the top of the shoulders, where we often hold tension. It is very warming and relaxing to receive, and can easily be self-applied too.

*Try single-handed kneading on another person's shoulders. Apply a little carrier oil to the shoulders, then place your fingers over the top of each shoulder so they are pointing toward the chest. Start to squeeze the muscles between the palm of your hand and your fingers, as though you were wringing out a cloth.*

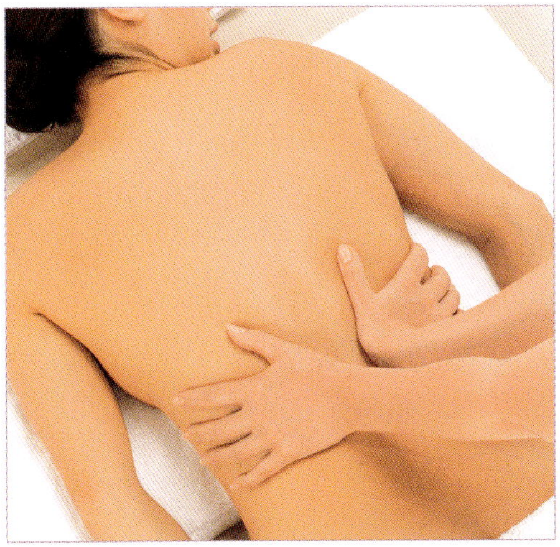

### FANNING

This is another variety of effleurage stroke which is very relaxing. It warms the area, and you can increase the pressure gradually, checking with the person you are working on that it feels good. Fanning encourages good circulation, and can be used on the back or the legs.

*Try fanning on someone else's back. Apply a little carrier oil to help your hands to help them move smoothly. Place both hands at the base of the spine, with your wrists together. Now squeeze in an outward direction, fanning the hands sideways; slowly move up the back toward the shoulders, then stroke back down to the base and start again.*

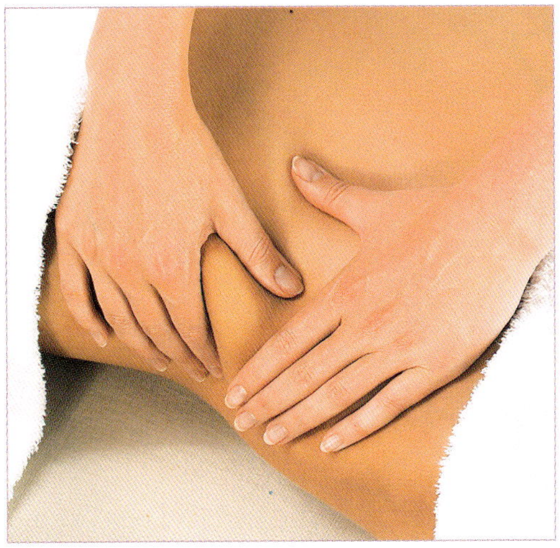

### DOUBLE-HANDED KNEADING

This movement is like kneading bread dough. It requires more co-ordination, but the key is to start very slowly. Kneading is an important massage stroke; it really stretches and compresses the muscle fibres, encouraging good circulation. Use it on areas such as the shoulders, waist, thighs and hips.

*Try double-handed kneading on the side of another person's abdomen. Apply a little carrier oil to your hands first, then pick up and squeeze the flesh between your thumb and fingers, first with one hand then the other, so you start an alternate rhythm, left and right.*

# basic massage strokes: 3

These strokes give more variation – some are more stimulating and some more calming. They are often combined with effleurage or kneading; for example, on very stiff shoulders you might alternate kneading with thumb pressures to ease tense muscles.

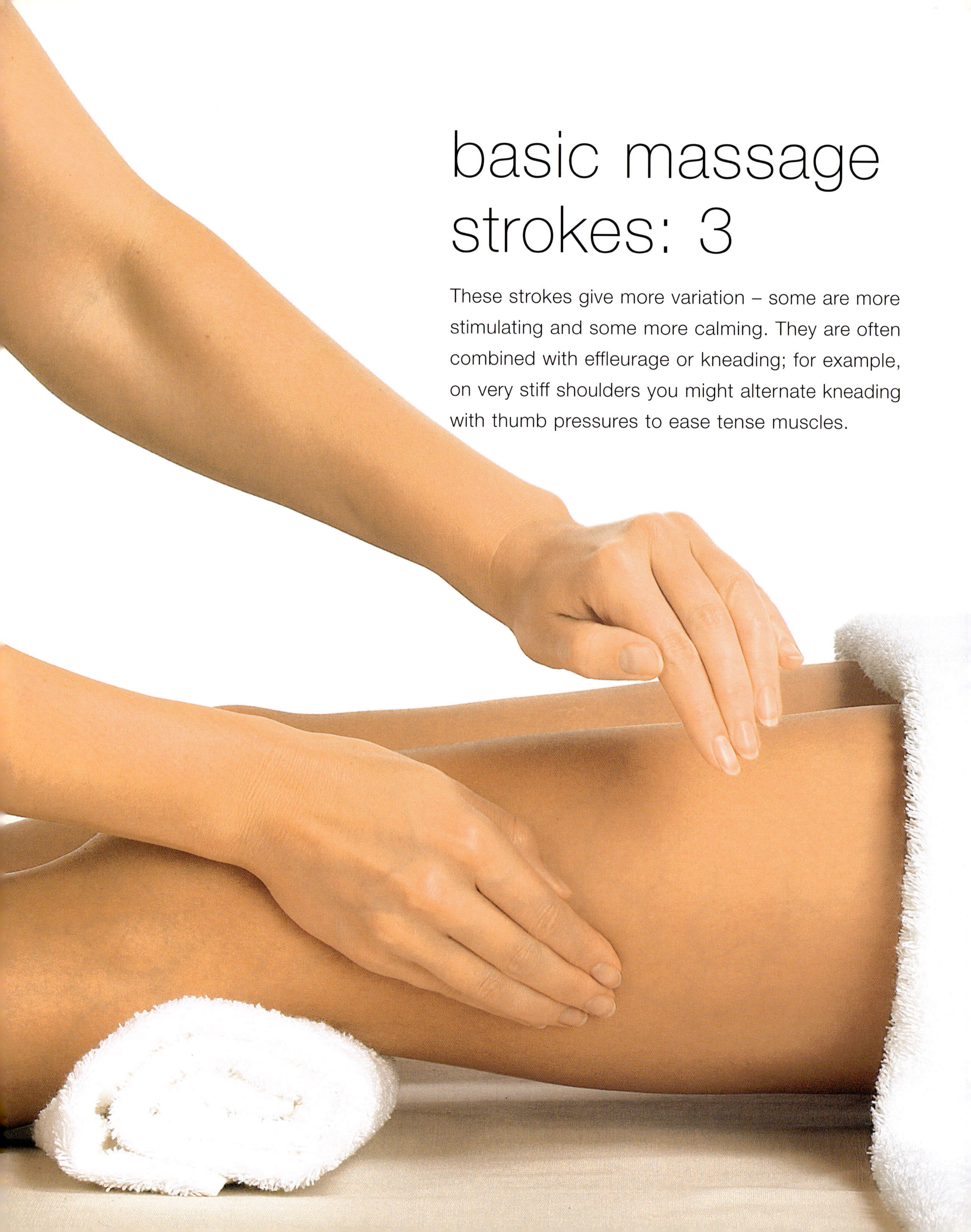

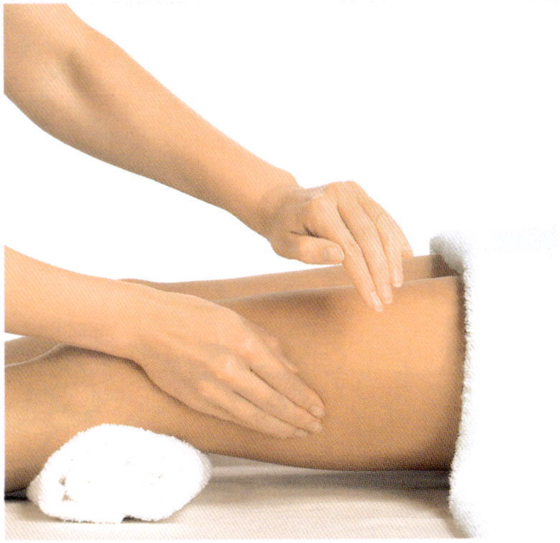

### CUPPING

This stroke is more stimulating, and helps to break down toxins as well as ease stiff muscle fibres. It feels brisk and light to receive. Use cupping on the thighs, hips or legs to help improve circulation.

*Try cupping on someone's thigh. Place your hands lightly together over the area, fingers loose and lightly touching each other, then using the edge of your hands, flick them alternately against the muscle in a light, fast rhythm. Keep your fingers relaxed and let your wrist do the work.*

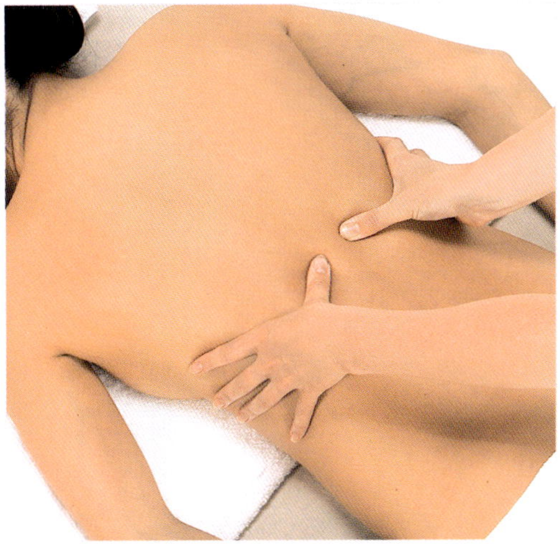

### THUMB PRESSURES

This is a much more localized movement, which is used on specific areas. To do it you should try to keep your thumbs as straight as possible, so you don't overstrain any of your thumb joints. Check with the recipient that they feel pressure, but no actual pain.

*Try this on another person's back. Start with the thumbs on either side of the spine at the base of the back, about 1in (2.5cm) apart. Lean on your thumbs, applying pressure for a few seconds, then ease off. Move upward about 1in (2.5cm), then repeat the pressure, and carry on all the way up the spine.*

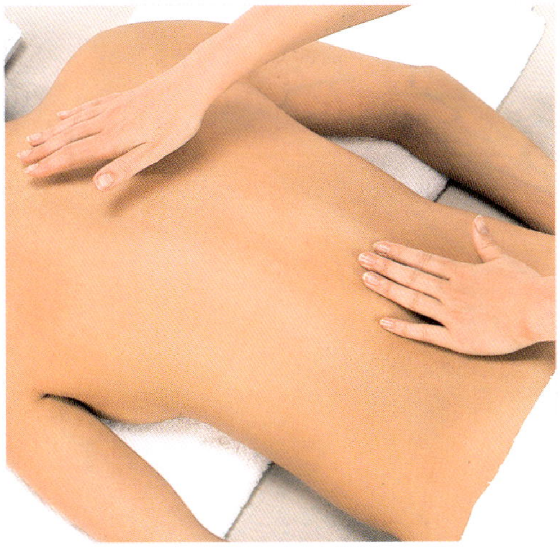

### REFLEX STROKE

This is a lovely stroke with which to end a treatment, particulary if you have done some thorough work on tense areas. It is an extremly light touch, but is a stroking movement and should not feel ticklish.

*Try this over someone else's spine. Simply glide the hands from shoulder level down to the hips, one after the other, as if you were stroking a cat. Practise this movement slowly and very smoothly. It is extremly relaxing to receive.*

# massage with essential oil

I am often asked, if massage alone is so powerful, why add essential oils to the treatment? My answer is that these oils add an amazing enhancement to a massage and, together, both tools create a new experience. Essential oils also have particular therapeutic effects, the most important of which are discussed below.

Once somebody who has given massage without essential oils experiences the effects of massage using oils, their work tends to remain aromatic! Different oils have a range of positive physical and psychological effects on both the giver and receiver of aromatherapy massage, which only increase the benefits of this holistic therapeutic treatment.

### INCREASED CIRCULATION

The essential oils rosemary, peppermint, cardamom, black pepper and ginger contain ingredients that have a stimulating effect on local circulation. Blends made with these essential oils have an immediate warming effect as they are applied, which the person receiving the massage experiences as a sense of tingling or heat. The person giving the massage may observe the effects either as heat under their hands, or as a spreading pink glow on the skin area above the muscle. This is quite normal. The person receiving should be able to feel improved movement, especially if an area has been stiff or sore. The advantages of using essential oils with these properties is that they speed up the process of relieving stiffness and pain so the person giving the massage does not have to work so hard to release a problem area. The effects of the treatment generally last for several hours after the massage has been given.

### TO FRAGRANCE OR NOT TO FRAGRANCE?

Try this exercise to see for yourself the difference made by adding essential oils to a massage treatment. Arrange to perform two massage treatments on a friend on consecutive days. You need to give the massage at the same time of day, in the same location, and must use identical massage movements (try the back routine; pp.54–57).

The first time you do your treatment, use a plain carrier oil with no essential oils in it at all. There should be no other fragrance in the room while you give the massage. As you work, assess your own energy levels. Do you feel energized or tired? Is the treatment easy or is it an effort? Ask your friend to describe their experience of the treatment and their mood at the end of it. You might like to make a few notes.

On the second occasion, make up this simple blend: in 20ml (4tsp) carrier oil (try grapeseed or sweet almond oil), add 4 drops of lavender and 6 drops of sweet orange essential oils. Then apply this blend to your friend using exactly the same massage movements as the day before. Notice again how it feels to give the treatment and if you feel tired or energized at the end. Ask your friend the same questions as the previous day, and discuss whether or not there was a difference between the two treatments. Did you both think the essential oils and their aroma made the second treatment more or less effective?

Try this exercise with several people and record the feedback you get. In terms of the results of your experiments, I leave that to you – I'm not going to try to influence you!

## INCREASED PAIN RELIEF

Sometimes it can be challenging to work on areas that the person receiving feels are tense and sore, because they may be slightly anxious that the treatment will be painful. Essential oils with pain-relieving and relaxing qualities, such as lavender, vetiver, German chamomile, yarrow and sweet marjoram, can be made into soothing blends that act quickly to calm and relax, and ease pain in aching areas. Applied with firm but soothing strokes – try effleurage and kneading – blends containing these oils will often make the person receiving fall fast asleep.

## POSITIVE PSYCHOLOGICAL EFFECTS

The aroma of whichever aromatherapy blend you use will have an effect on the person receiving treatment. As soon as the massage starts, the action of applying the blend to the skin spreads the aroma into the room. Some essential oils such as grapefruit, sweet orange, frankincense, rose, neroli and mandarin have directly uplifting and cheering effects on the mind, because they are the fruit and flowers of summertime and the associations here are so often positive. Adding oils like these to blends always brings a sense of freshness and lightness, improving moods and feelings.

Remember, too, that the aroma of the blend used is also perceived by the person giving the massage and the fragrance also affects them, though not as strongly as it does the person receiving. This rather subtle effect helps the person giving to feel more energized while performing the treatment and also makes it easier for them to do a couple of sessions back to back. Aromatherapists often feel that the energetic qualities of any essential oils they use help to keep them going while they do several treatments. Even if the oils being used have calming properties, the aroma itself helps the practitioner to maintain concentration.

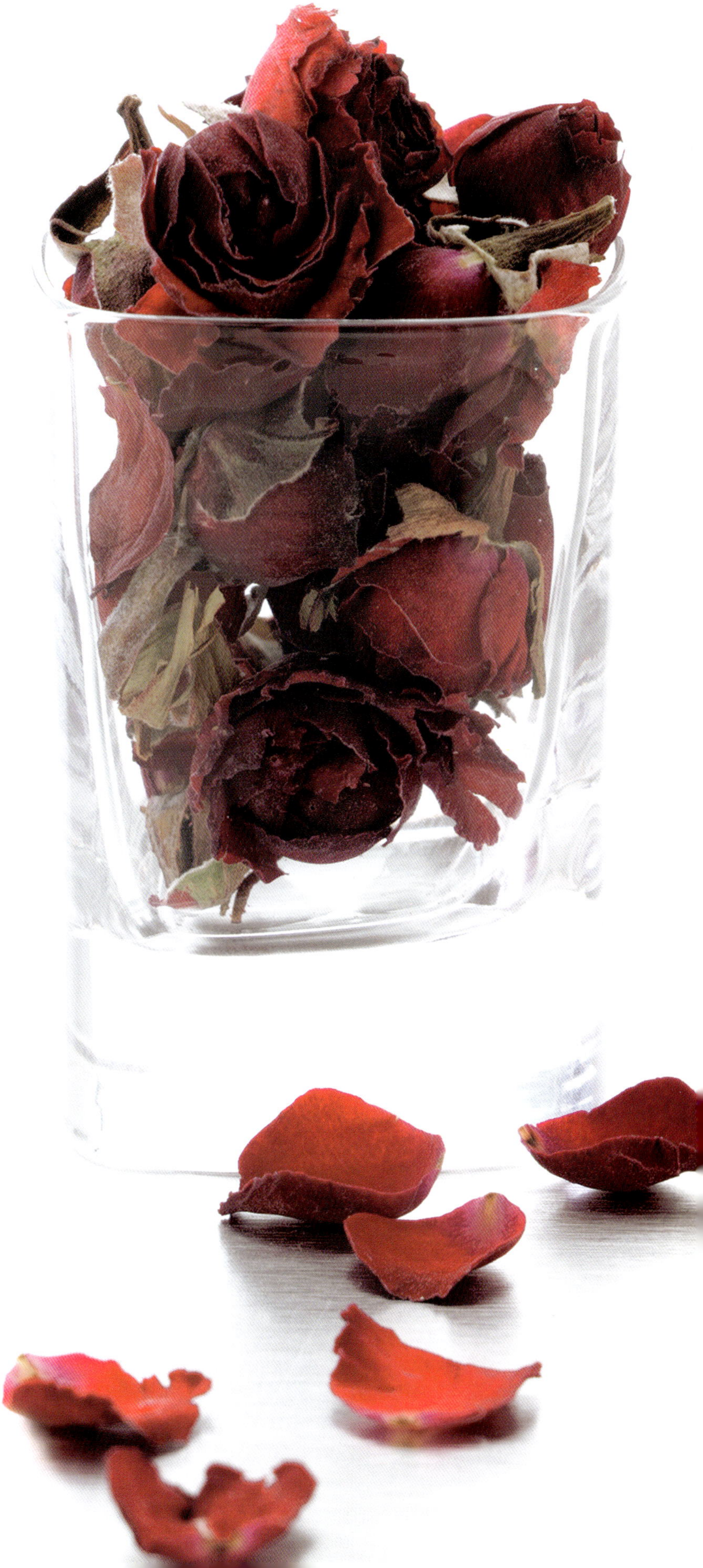

# massage as an exchange

Massage is, by its very nature, a form of intimate communication with another person. It involves understanding and trust, and so it is very important to be aware of the more personal aspects of the exchange between the giver and the receiver.

Massage is not something everyone has experienced. I still meet people who have never had a treatment and have no idea what it entails. One of the most common misconceptions is that you have to undress completely, and this can put off many people. In some northern European countries there can be quite strong levels of reserve, especially among the more mature age groups, and this means you need to put people at ease. I always explain that towels are draped over you to keep you warm during the treatment, and that only the area being worked on at any time is left exposed. This is particularly important to stress if you are going to massage someone who is perhaps a friend or an acquaintance rather than a close family member.

The oldest client I ever worked on was a glorious elderly lady in her mid-eighties; she would tell me wonderful stories of her youth while I massaged her back, neck and shoulders. At first she was very unsure about

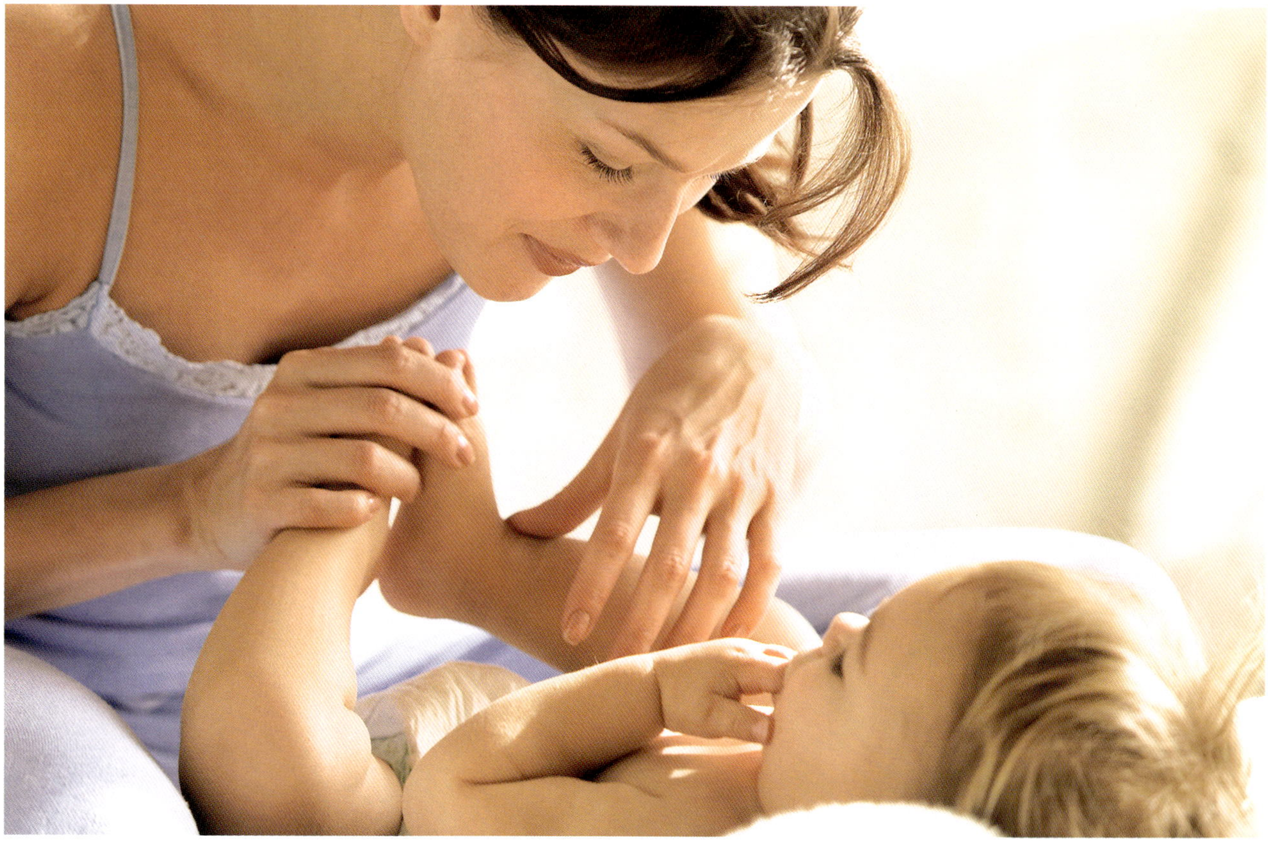

undressing in front of me and was worried about my seeing her body. I reassured her by working on her hands and feet first, until she got used to me, and when she realized that I was in no way judging how she looked, she let me work on her back.

I find the human body astonishing, no matter what a person's age, size or shape. It is very gratifying to see how positive a person can become about themselves through the experience of respectful touch.

## WORKING WITH RESPECT

If you work on someone and they are totally happy with what you are doing, they will get the maximum benefit from the massage and you will know you have given a worthwhile treatment. Here are some guidelines to help inform your work.

### Personal boundaries

We all have boundaries – things we will accept or not accept. Because of the level of trust needed during massage, it is important to respect how the person receiving may feel about aspects of the treatment. Some people hate their feet being touched, and others feel very unsure about abdominal massage. If there is any part of the body that the person receiving does not want you to treat, it is important to respect this. You may find that as you work more often with them this attitude changes, but it is not a good idea to try to force anyone to accept treatment they may not want.

### Cultural considerations

Although massage is common to many cultures in the world, it is also common to find different attitudes toward it. For example, in some cultures the giver and the receiver have to be the same sex. If you treat someone with a particular cultural attitude toward massage, simply work as the person receiving asks and is able to accept.

### Working with minors

In many cultures, massage is given across age groups, but only between family members. Using massage with babies and young children is very beneficial for their sleeping or tummy problems, and older children can find it helps reduce stress. I have many aromatherapist colleagues whose offspring have grown up with massage and for whom it is a totally natural thing to receive. However, massage must always be given with consent, and if you are asked to work on someone under the age of 16, a parent or a guardian should always be present.

### Developing your awareness and getting feedback

As you gain in confidence by massaging friends and family, you will develop your own awareness of what others need. The more you practise particular techniques, the more your hands will communicate how the recipient is feeling – for example, whether they are comfortable, or tense and ill at ease. Some people pick up these signals quickly; others take longer. It is good to talk to your recipient to get feedback during treatment. If they express discomfort always slow down, release pressure and work gently until they feel better. The more relaxed the recpient is during treatment, the easier it is for you to release aches, pains and tense muscles.

### Looking after yourself

It is common to become so enthusiastic about giving massage that you forget to take care of yourself. Because the emphasis is on the recipient, you forget your own posture or push yourself to give a treatment when you are tired. This is not helpful. Be aware that when you perform a massage you expend energy. This is especially true when you are learning – you may find it quite tiring. It is therefore important to pace yourself. Never push yourself too far. It's far better to do a little work regularly than a lot of work in one go.

# setting up your massage space

If you are going to give a really relaxing massage treatment, you need to prepare a space to work in. Few of us have a special treatment room in our own home, but with a little attention it is possible to turn any space into an area suitable for massage.

Here are some ideas to think about when you set up your massage space. It helps to imagine how you would like to feel yourself if you were receiving a treatment.

**ENVIRONMENT**

This means the whole area dedicated to massage and everything in it. Your space needs to be tidy, clutter-free and clean, partly for hygiene reasons but also because this creates a more restful atmosphere for the recipient. Switch off all phones and keep any pets elsewhere while you work. If you are working in the evening, use soft, subdued lighting. Candles are ideal, but be sure to place them somewhere safe. Some people like to play soothing music while they work; others prefer quiet. I like to work with soft classical music in the background.

**ROOM TEMPERATURE**

This is crucial! When we start to relax, our body temperature drops by a few degrees. The recipient needs to be kept warm while you work, so you may find that you need to increase the heating. This might make you hot, but it is vitally important that the recipient is able to relax – an impossible task if they are cold.

**MASSAGE SURFACE**

Professional massage therapists and aromatherapists work on special massage treatment tables. However, these are expensive to buy. You are most likely to be giving a treatment on the floor, and for this the best surface is a thick, double futon mattress. This will allow the recipient to lie comfortably and also enable you to kneel beside them without hurting your knees. An alternative would be to buy a piece of thick foam rubber cut to size; you would need a square 6ft (2m) long by 6ft (2m) wide. Spread a thick blanket over the surface of your mattress or foam pad and, over that, a clean cotton sheet for the recipent to lie on. It is also helpful to have three flat, oblong pillows to hand to prop up their knees or for them to rest their head on comfortably.

**TOWELS AND ARRANGEMENT**

It is best to buy some large thick towels that you keep purely for massage purposes. They will need to be laundered in very hot water to get rid of any carrier oil stains so they must be made from 100 per cent cotton pile. Four bath-size towels should be sufficient for one massage. The simplest towel arrangement is to lay one towel horizontally across the top part of the body, and a second towel lengthways down the legs. Then you simply move a section aside at a time to work on the limbs. The other towels can be rolled up as leg, arm or neck supports as you need them. If the recipent feels chilly, you may need to lay a light blanket over the top while you work. This is very warm and comforting.

### HYGIENE

Aromatherapy massage is more effective if the recipient has a shower immediately before the session – research has shown that essential oils and carriers penetrate the skin better if it is very slightly damp and soft. Wash your own hands before and after giving a treatment. Also, have some disposable wet wipes available, for example to wipe the recipient's feet before working on them.

### WHAT YOU SHOULD WEAR

The best clothing to wear for giving a massage is a loose cotton T-shirt and cotton trousers such as leggings, or a light tracksuit. You will tend to get warm while you work, so breathable cotton is preferable to manmade fibres. Make sure that you can move easily in your chosen clothes – if they are too tight your movements will be restricted.

### MATERIALS

Before you start working, gather together your essential oils, your carrier oil and your blend bottle. Measure out the carrier oil – then all that you need to do is to add the right number of drops of essential oil to make your blend. Set up your materials on a tray on a low table so that you can reach them easily and wipe up any spills. You will need to discuss with the recipient what effect – for example, relaxing or energizing – they would like the massage to have, and what type of scent they prefer (so you will need all your essential oils to hand, too). I like to keep mine together in a special wooden box. It's good to give the recipient an idea of the overall aroma of the blend before you make it. I usually take the tops off the relevant bottles, hold them together and let the person smell the tiny amount of essential oil inside the lids. This gives a fair approximation of the scent you will make.

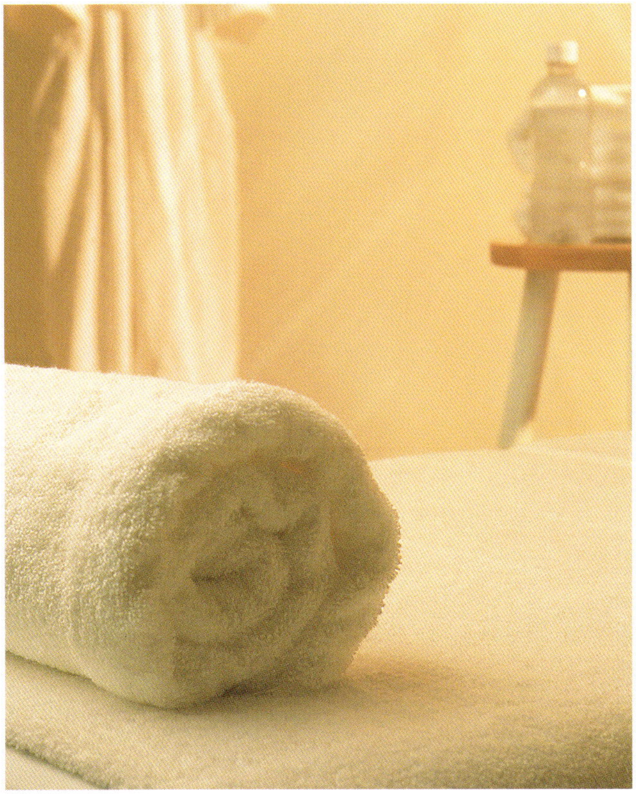

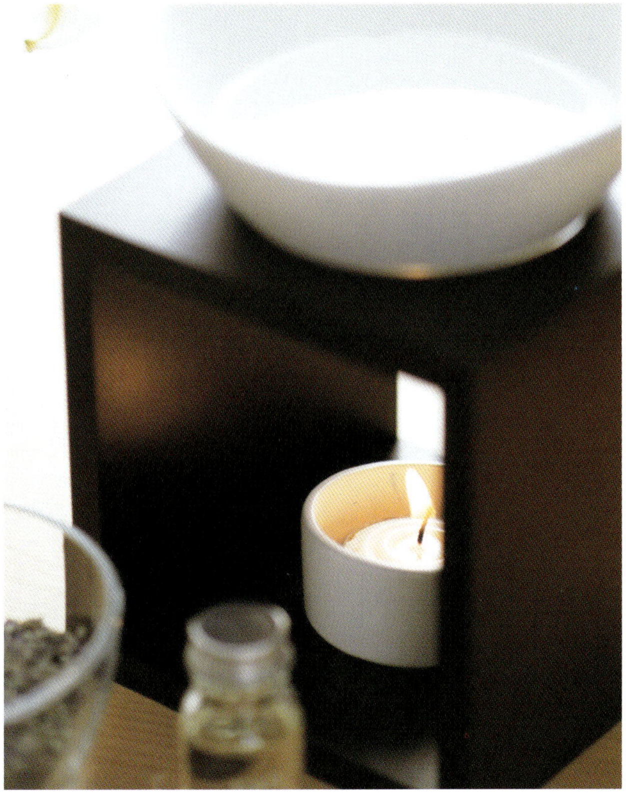

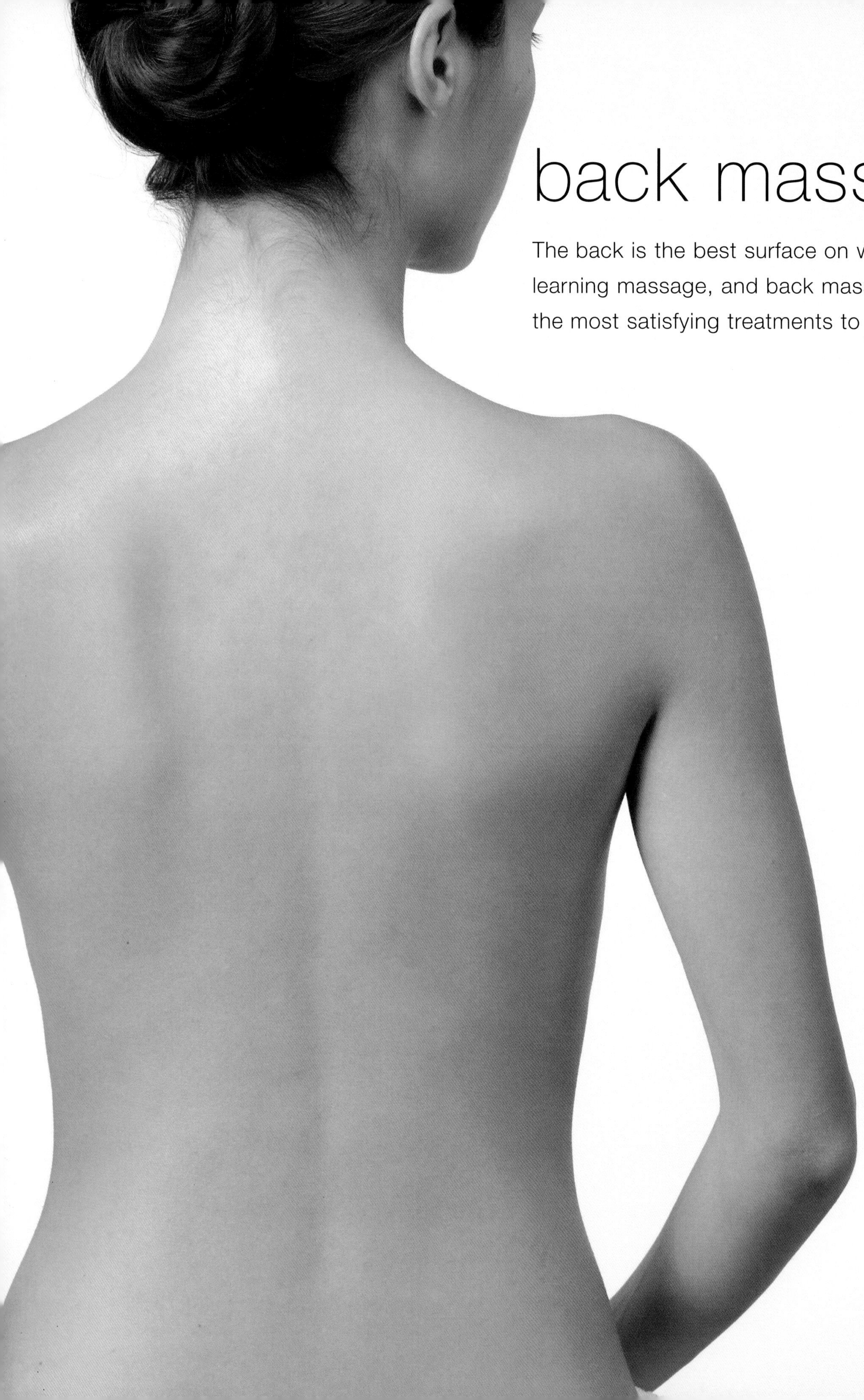

# back massage

The back is the best surface on which to start learning massage, and back massage is one of the most satisfying treatments to give and receive.

As the back is such a large area, it enables you to practise your massage movements easily. For the person receiving, especially if they are unfamiliar with massage, the back is a non-threatening area to have treated, and one that responds quickly to caring touch. Back aches and stiffness are extremely common, especially because so many of us lead sedentary lives and maintain poor posture while sitting at work. Companies spend a huge amount of money each year on sickness pay for employees with back pain or back troubles. Regular back massage really can help to keep such problems at bay.

### THE STRUCTURE OF THE BACK

The back consists of three main parts, the first of which is the spine itself. This is the bony ridge that runs from the base of the skull all the way down to the coccyx, or tailbone, between the buttocks. Second are the bones of the shoulder blades and pelvic girdle, which are attached to the top of the spine and to the sacrum at the base of the back respectively. The last part consists of the major groups of muscles attached to the bones of the back, which allow us to move and lift things, and help support our bodies while we undertake our daily activities.

The spine itself is made up of individual bones called vertebrae, held apart by soft pads of spinal disks. The whole spine is very mobile; seen from the side it sits naturally in a gentle S-shaped curve. The vertebrae divide into five groups: the seven small cervical vertebrae in the neck; the 12 larger thoracic vertebrae in the upper trunk; the five lumbar vertebrae in the lower back – these are very strong and bear our weight; the sacrum – a triangular-shaped bony area at the base of the spine, attached to the pelvic girdle; and the coccyx, made of tiny vertebrae, which curls up between the buttocks.

The main muscle groups you will be massaging are in the shoulders, down the sides of the spine and at the base of the spine. The trapezius is the large diamond-shaped muscle that is attached at the top to the base of the skull and the shoulders, and which runs all the way down to the middle of the back. The latissimus dorsi muscles lie on the left and right sides of the torso, from just under the armpit to just above the top curve of the hip area. And the gluteus maximus muscles are found at the very base of the back and over the buttock area.

### BACK MASSAGE SAFETY CHECK

Before you start any treatment, ask the person who wishes to receive the massage a few simple questions to assess whether or not it is advisable to proceed. Do they have a viral illness such as a cold or flu? If yes, don't work. Do they have any recent injuries affecting the back area? If yes and these are severe, don't work. Do they have any problem areas in the back? If yes and these are severe, don't work; if there is just general stiffness or muscular aches, it is fine to go ahead. Finally, in the case of pregnancy, the intended receiver may not feel comfortable lying on her front, and may prefer to lie on her side propped up with pillows; also check if her midwife is happy for her to receive massage, and remember to halve the number of stated drops of essential oils in your blend (see pp.26–27).

### SETTING UP YOUR TREATMENT

Place a blanket and then a clean cotton sheet on your futon or foam mat. The receiver needs to lie face down, with their head propped up on a flat pillow or a folded towel. An extra folded towel under the shins may give additional comfort. Cover their back with a large towel laid horizontally across, and their legs with a towel laid lengthwise. Put a light blanket over the whole body to start with, so that their body becomes warm, then fold the upper towel back over the legs, tucking it into their underwear before you begin.

# BACK MASSAGE ROUTINE: 1

These are warming strokes to get the area ready for deeper work. Choose your blend and make it up ready to use. Kneel next to the receiver's hips, on their right side. If you need more padding under your knees, use a folded towel. The recipient should rest their head on a flat pillow, but may turn the head if it becomes uncomfortable to stay in one position. Try to keep your own back straight while you work. If you forget what to do next at any time, just carry on stroking as you pick up the next step!

**SUGGESTED BACK MASSAGE BLENDS**

There are a wide variety of essential oils that can be combined together for a back massage. Blends can be tailored to suit the particular needs of the intended recipient on any given day. I have divided the blends into groups that have similar effects on the mind and body, and have given suggestions for the best times of day at which to apply them.

| | WHEN TO USE | BLENDS |
|---|---|---|
| RELAXING AND CALMING BLENDS | These blends are particularly good for evening treatments. All are relaxing and soothing in pregnancy but remember to use half the stated number of essential oil drops in the full amount of carrier oil. | *In 4tsp (20ml) carrier oil (sweet almond, grapeseed or jojoba):*<br>• Lavender 4 drops, Mandarin 4 drops, Sandalwood 2 drops<br>• Geranium 2 drops, Rosewood 4 drops, Lemon 4 drops<br>• Neroli 2 drops, Sweet orange 6 drops, Petitgrain 2 drops |
| INVIGORATING AND CIRCULATION-STIMULATING BLENDS | These blends are good for morning or daytime treatments. They help alleviate aches and pains, but contain ingredients that are too mentally stimulating to use in the evening. | *In 4tsp (20ml) carrier oil (grapeseed, camellia or jojoba):*<br>• Black pepper 2 drops, Rosemary 4 drops, Juniper 4 drops<br>• Nutmeg 2 drops, Lemongrass 2 drops, Grapefruit 6 drops<br>• Peppermint 2 drops, Lemon 6 drops, Spanish sage 2 drops |
| MUSCLE-WARMING AND SOOTHING BLENDS | These blends are especially good for evening treatments. They ease aches and pains and will encourage restful sleep. | *In 4tsp (20ml) carrier oil (sweet almond, grapeseed or avocado):*<br>• Lavender 6 drops, Vetiver 2 drops, Ginger 2 drops<br>• German chamomile 2 drops, Lavendin 4 drops, Carrot seed 4 drops<br>• Cardamom 4 drops, Coriander seed 4 drops, May chang 2 drops |
| UPLIFTING AND MOOD-ENHANCING BLENDS | These blends are exotic and uplifting combinations which have positive effects on mood. They are suitable for treatments at any time of the day or evening. | *In 4tsp (20ml) carrier oil (apricot kernel, jojoba or sweet almond):*<br>• Ylang ylang 2 drops, Mandarin 4 drops, Rosewood 4 drops<br>• Sandalwood 2 drops, Frankincense 4 drops, Grapefruit 4 drops<br>• Sweet orange 6 drops, Patchouli 2 drops, Rose 2 drops |

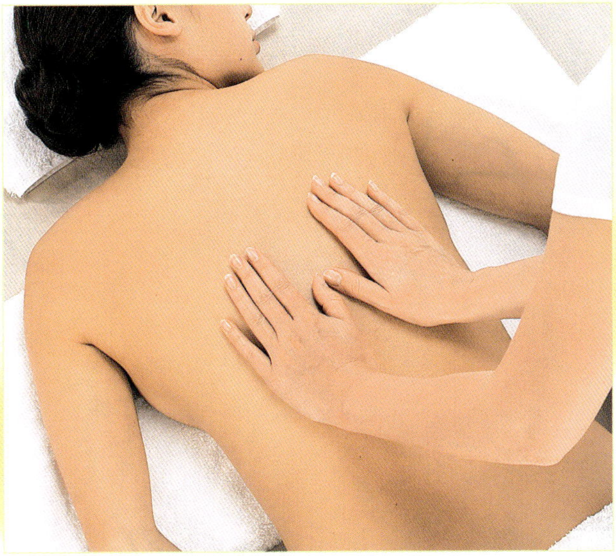

**1. Effleurage:** Pour a teaspoon of blend into your hands, rub them together gently and place them parallel to each other at the base of the back, either side of the spine. Stroke all the way up the back, across the shoulders, down the sides and return to where you started. Repeat this stroke with light pressure several times to warm the back.

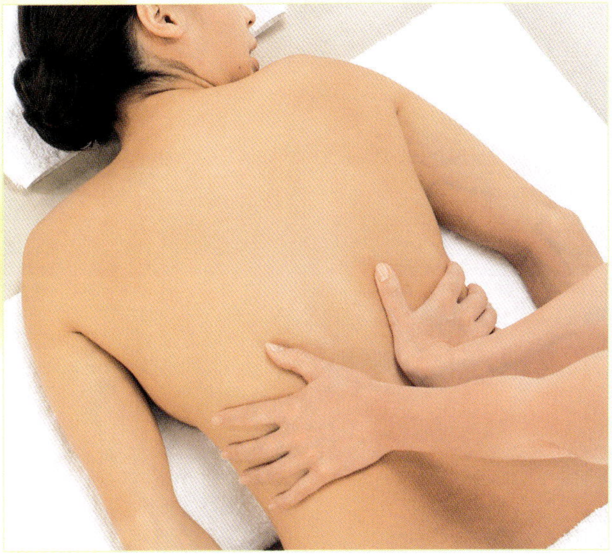

**2. Fanning:** Start with both hands at the base of the spine, fingers spread out and wrists together. Fan the hands out toward the sides of the back, applying quite firm pressure. Bring them back to centre and repeat the stroke three times over the lower back, three times over the mid back and three times over the shoulder area.

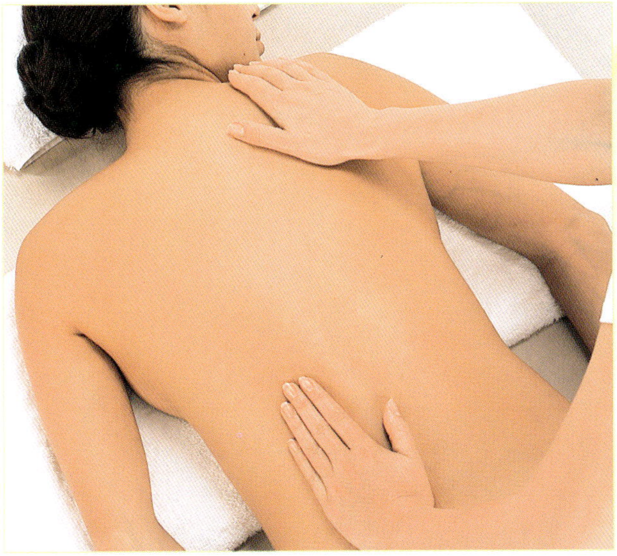

**3. Alternate stroking:** Start with your right hand on the recipient's right shoulder, and your left hand just above their left hip. Stroke all the way up and down the sides of the back with your hands moving in opposite directions. Repeat several times.

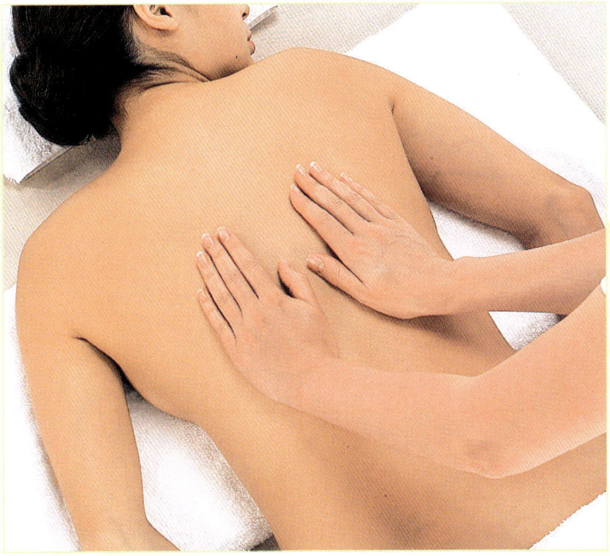

4. Repeat the effleurage stroke (see step 1), but this time apply more definite pressure, up the back, out over the shoulders, down the sides and return to the starting position. You should really be able to feel the skin warming under your hands.

# BACK MASSAGE ROUTINE: 2

Here you will be working more deeply into areas which may hold some tension or stiffness. Always check that the recipient feels happy with the pressure you are using; they should tell you if anything is uncomfortable. In any tender areas, ease off the pressure at first, then increase it again gradually.

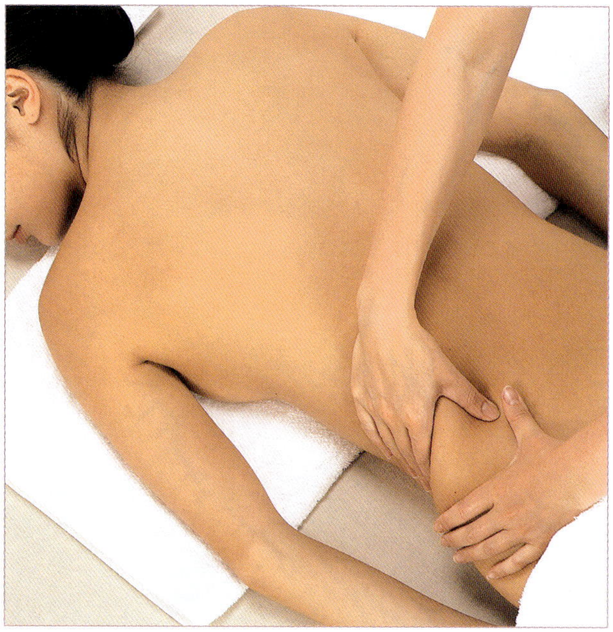

1. **Kneading:** Use this stroke on the sides of the body. Stay kneeling on the right-hand side of the receiver's body, facing across their torso. Start kneading up and down that side of the torso from the buttock and hip up toward the armpit, really squeezing and wringing the flesh; then transfer your hands to the side of the torso nearest to you and repeat kneading there.

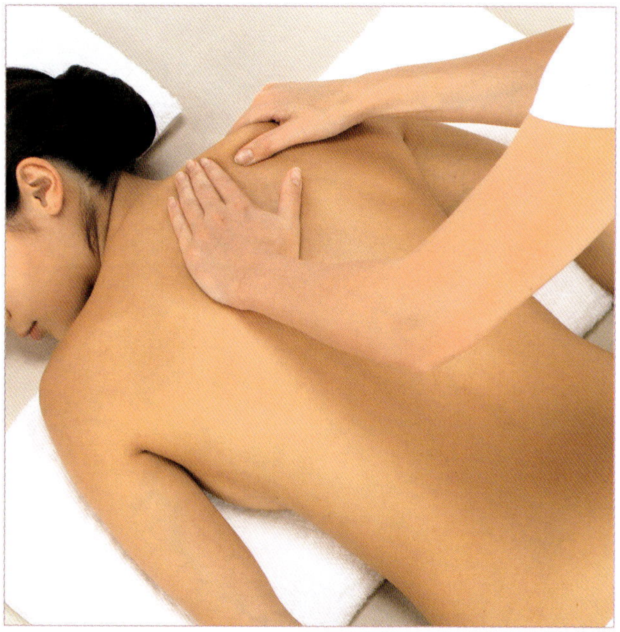

2. **Shoulder kneading:** Next, move up to kneel by the waist, still on the right side. Use both hands to knead into the muscles at the top of the shoulders, starting gently then increasing pressure gradually. If you find double-handed kneading too difficult, use one hand on each shoulder and try single-handed kneading.

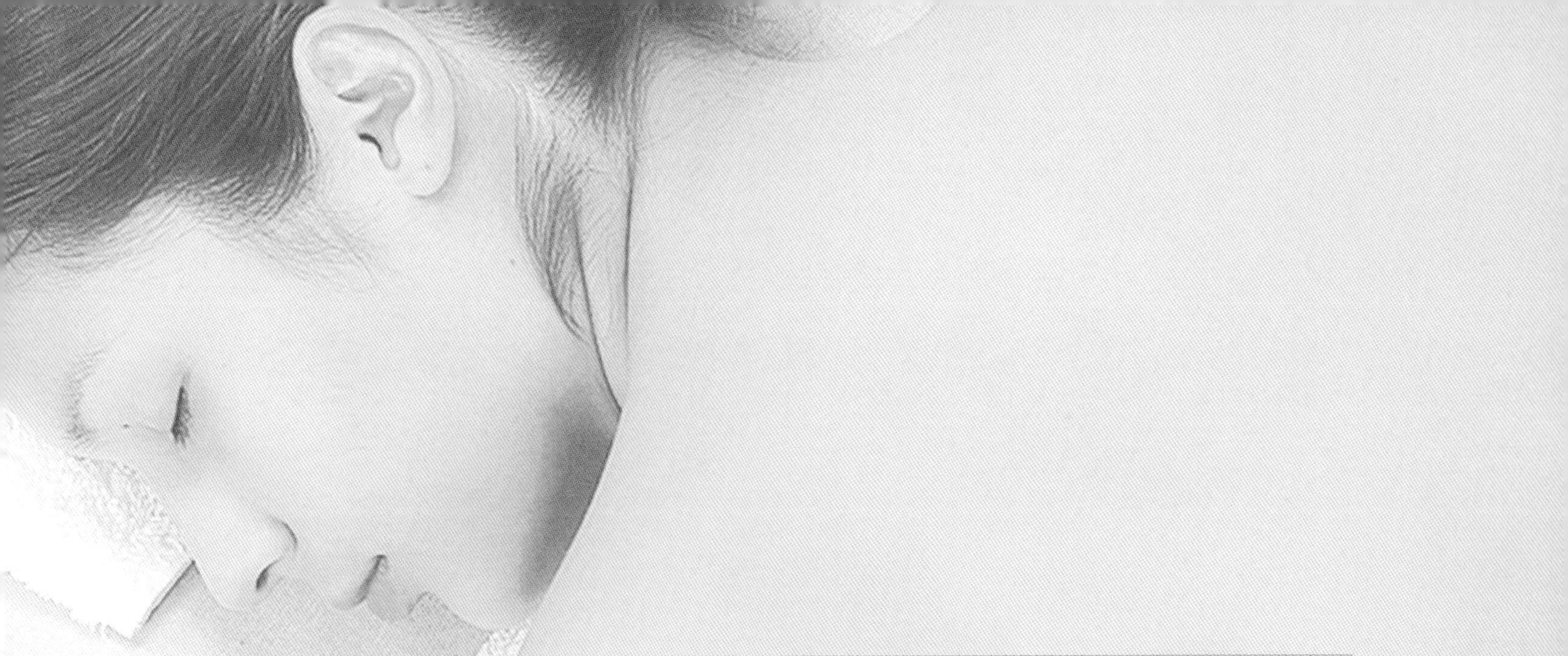

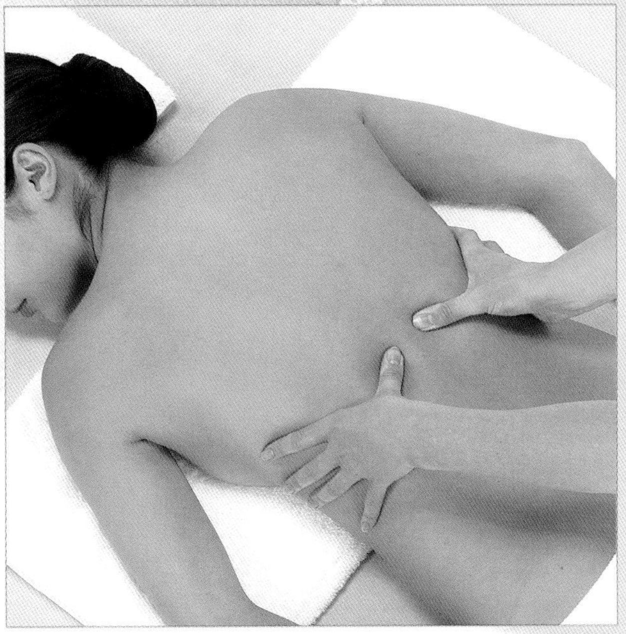

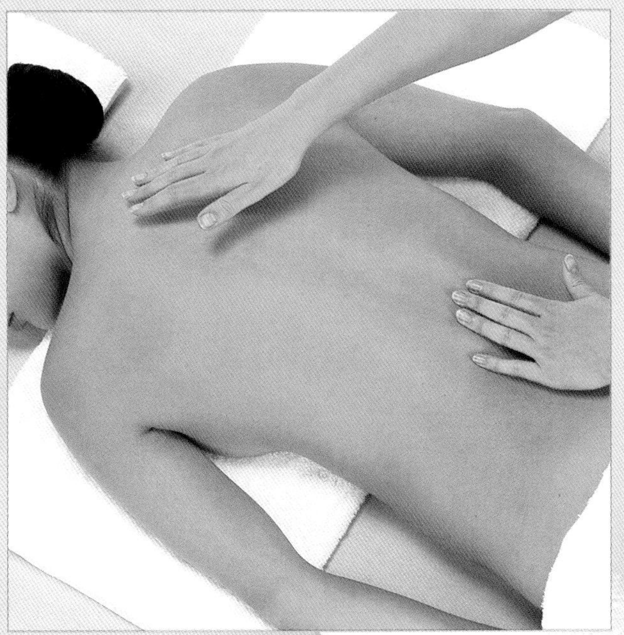

**3. Thumb pressures:** Move back to kneel just by the receiver's right hip. Place both thumbs on either side of the base of the spine – there is a groove you will be able to feel just next to the vertebrae. Gently lean on your thumbs to apply pressure for a few seconds, then move up a little way, and repeat the pressures. Continue until you have travelled all the way up the spine.

**4. Reflex strokes:** Place both hands at the top of the shoulders and start stroking down the back smoothly and gently, one hand following the other. This will calm the area as you finish your massage. Let your reflex strokes become slower and slower, until you glide very gently off the back to end.

Finally, re-cover the person receiving the massage with the towel and put a blanket overf them to keep them warm. Allow them to rest for a while and to inhale the aroma of the blend you have just massaged into their body.

# neck and shoulder massage

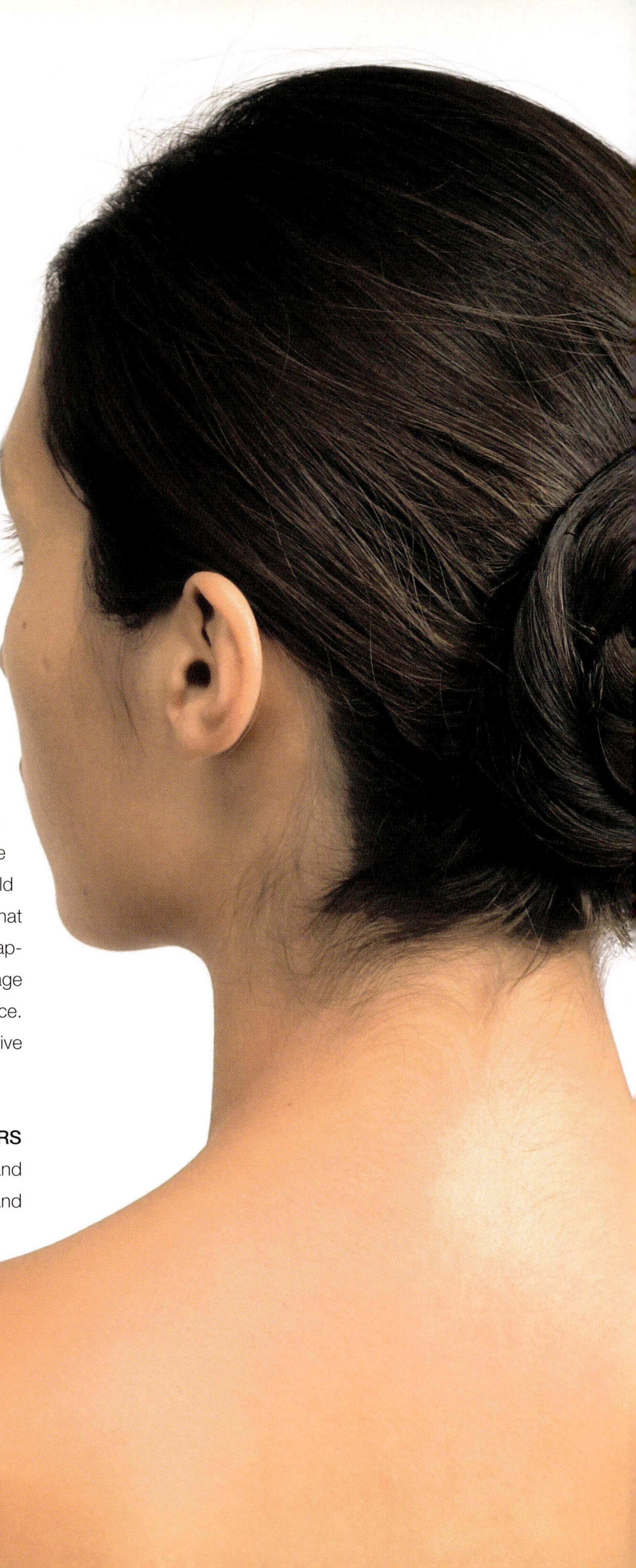

The neck and shoulder area is a common sites of tension and discomfort in the body. Much of this results from our sedentary lifestyles and poor posture, which increase the strain on the muscles.

Many people come for professional aromatherapy treatment complaining of neck and shoulder pain. Often this has a physical cause, such as poor posture, but it may also have some links to emotional stress. Hunching and curving of the shoulders can be seen as a kind of self-protection, and many people hold their anxiety and stress in this area. You may find that massage releases some of these feelings. If this happens simply cover up the person receiving the massage and sit with them so that you are a reassuring presence. This is all you are required to be. The relaxation you give them through the massage will be highly beneficial.

**THE STRUCTURE OF THE NECK AND SHOULDERS**

The neck supports the weight of the head – the skull and the brain inside it – which is about 10lbs (5kgs), and accounts for eight per cent of the body's total weight. The seven cervical vertebrae (see p.53) perform some of this supportive function, helped by complex groups of postural muscles which hold up the head and enable us to turn it from left to right and move it up and down. All the muscles in the neck area have to work hard to support the head, which is why they are often tired or tense at the end of the day. Awkward postures – such as cradling a telephone under one ear while doing something else – place extra stress on the neck and add considerably to its workload.

The neck connects with the shoulder bones – these are the collar bones at the front and the shoulder blades at the back – and from there is linked to the arms. Again, complex groups of muscles are involved here, allowing the arms and the torso to work together to help us to move flexibly, lift, push and pull in all the ways we need. If the neck area is tense, this can affect the arms and the middle of the back as we acquire bad postural habits to try to accommodate the area of discomfort. Regular neck and shoulder massage can help to keep the whole area supple and free from tension.

### NECK AND SHOULDER MASSAGE SAFETY CHECK

Before you start any treatment, ask the person who wishes to receive the massage a few simple questions to assess whether or not it is advisable to proceed. Do they have any injuries in the neck and shoulder area? If yes, don't work and refer the person to a medical professional. Are there any areas they describe as particularly tense or painful? If yes, and the discomfort is severe, it is better not to work; if the pain is minor to moderate in intensity, it is fine to proceed. Do they have a headache or migraine? If yes, do not work as massage in this area can make the person feel worse.

| SUGGESTED NECK AND SHOULDER MASSAGE BLENDS | | |
|---|---|---|
| | WHEN TO USE | BLENDS |
| RELAXING AND EMOTIONALLY-CALMING BLENDS | These blends are all good for evening work. They are relaxing and soothing in pregnancy but remember to use half the stated number of essential oil drops in the full amount of carrier oil. | *In 4tsp (20ml) carrier oil (sweet almond, grapeseed or jojoba):*<br>• Palmarosa 2 drops, Lemon 6 drops, Patchouli 2 drops<br>• Neroli 2 drops, Roman chamomile 2 drops, Sweet orange 6 drops<br>• Rose 2 drops, Mandarin 4 drops, Frankincense 4 drops |
| INVIGORATING AND CIRCULATION-STIMULATING BLENDS | These are powerful essential oils whose effects are particularly suitable for daytime work. They are far less suitable for evening treatments as some of the oils have strong mentally stimulating properties. | *In 4tsp (20ml) carrier oil (grapeseed or sweet almond):*<br>• Cumin seed 4 drops, Ginger 4 drops, Lemongrass 2 drops<br>• Rosemary 4 drops, Scotch pine 2 drops, Cypress 4 drops<br>• Juniper 2 drops, Spanish sage 4 drops, Lavendin 4 drops |
| SOOTHING AND MUSCLE-WARMING BLENDS | These blends are ideal for evening work as they are full of warming and spicy aromas which do wonders to relax both body and mind at the end of a hard day. | *In 4tsp (20ml) carrier oil (apricot kernel, jojoba or macadamia nut):*<br>• Carrot seed 4 drops, Vetiver 2 drops, Cardamom 4 drops<br>• Nutmeg 2 drops, Mandarin 4 drops, Coriander seed 4 drops<br>• Ginger 2 drops, Myrtle 6 drops, May chang 2 drops |

# NECK AND SHOULDER ROUTINE

To set up your treatment, place a thick blanket and cotton sheet on you futon mattress or foam mat. Invite the receiver to lie on their back, and place a flat pillow or rolled up towel under their knees to bend the legs a little. This helps to relax and release the lower back so that the person is more comfortable. Put a flat pillow under their head to support it while you work on the neck and shoulders. Place a large towel horizontally across the top of the body and cover the legs with a light blanket to keep them warm during the massage. Kneel above their head, perhaps with an extra pillow to support your knees. Be aware of your own posture while working, and keep your back as straight as you can. Choose one of the suggested neck and shoulder blends and make it up ready to use. Make sure your friend is comfortable on the mattress, then fold back the towel to just above their chest area while you work.

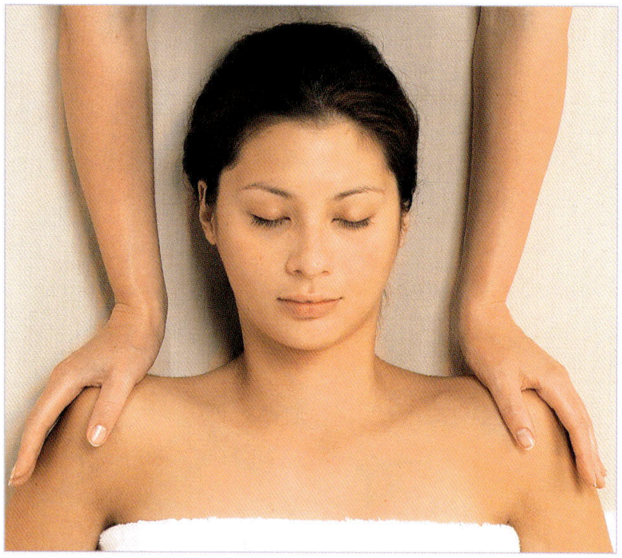

1. **Effleurage:** Take a teaspoon or two of your blend in your hands. Stroke it onto the skin, starting from the edges of the shoulders, over the top of the shoulders, up the back of the neck, back down and out to the sides. Repeat this stroke several times.

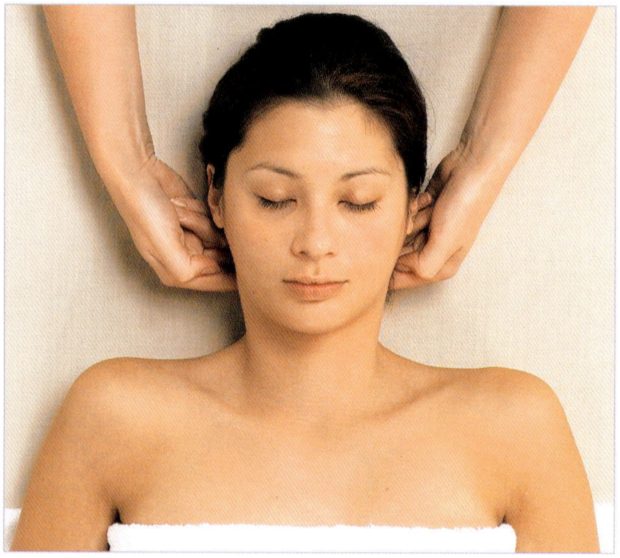

4. **Fingertip circles up the sides of the neck:** Place the fingertips of your index and middle fingers on either side of the base of the neck; feel them sit on either side of the vertebrae. Make tiny circles up the side of the neck into the hairline and gently stroke down. Repeat this several times.

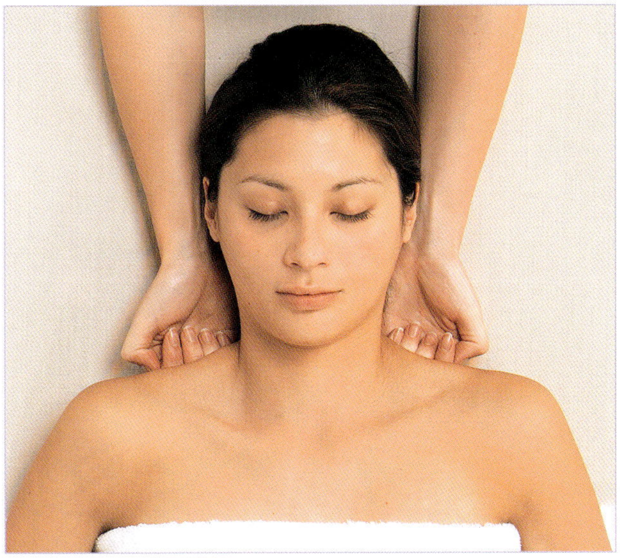

2. **Knuckling:** Next, knuckle all over the tops of the shoulders, up and down the back of the neck, and across the top of the chest. Repeat this series of movements until the area feels very warm and is glowing.

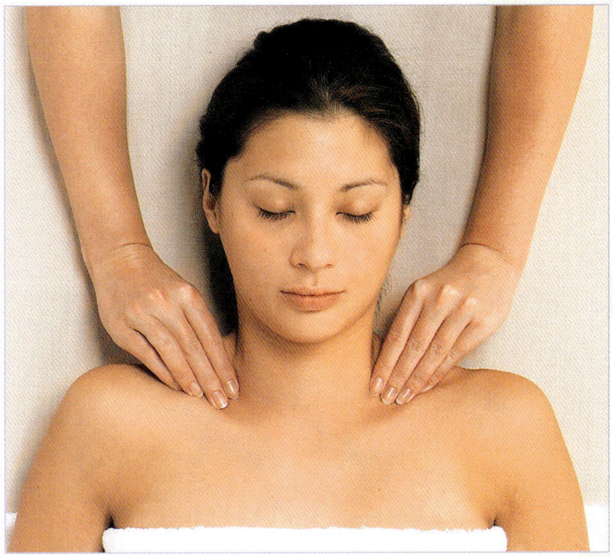

3. **Single-handed kneading:** With one hand on either side of the neck, knead the muscles at the tops of the shoulders, gently and slowly at first, increasing pressure as you continue. Check with the recipient that it feels good.

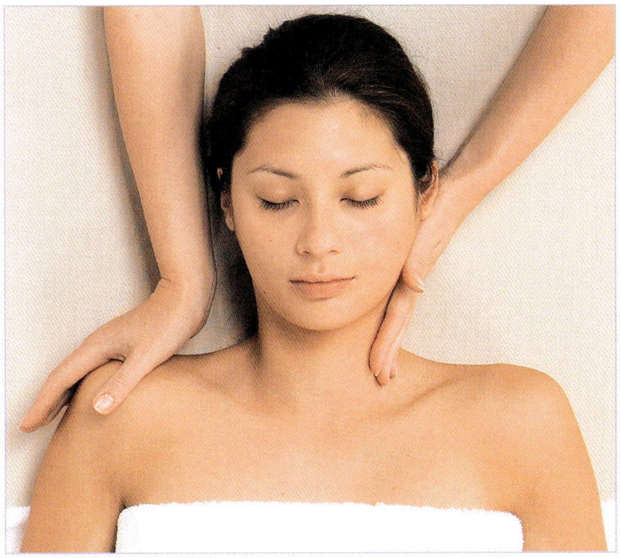

5. **Alternate deep stroking:** Place one hand on the side of each shoulder. Slowly stroke across the top of the shoulder and up the neck with firm pressure in one sweeping movement. Glide back with a lighter pressure, first with your left hand then your right. Repeat several times.

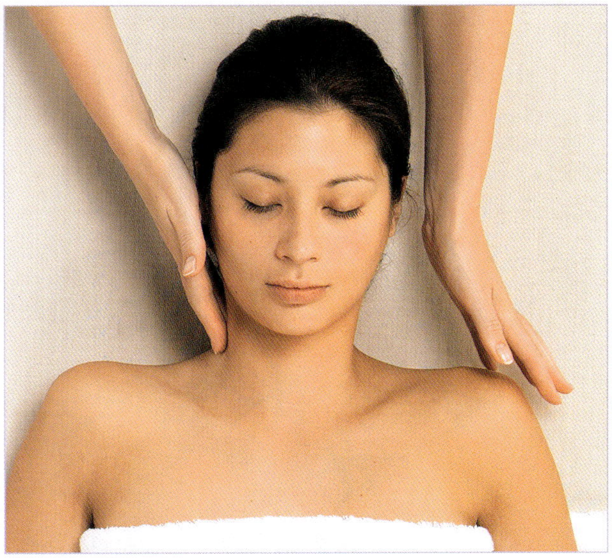

6. **Reflex strokes:** This is a continuation of the alternate stroking technique, except that your pressure on the upward sweep should become lighter and lighter until you glide gently off the neck to finish.

# face and décolletage massage

After practising routines on areas of the body such as the back and shoulders, which are covered by larger muscles, it is a totally different experience to work on an area like the face, where the musculature is on a much smaller scale.

You have been using the whole of the palm of your hand for most of your massage movements so far, but when you treat the face it is the fingertips that do most of the work because the movements required are tiny and need to be precise. Also, for the face and décolletage area both the carrier oils and the blends of essential oils have been specially selected to nourish and rejuvenate the skin. The blends are simpler and contain fewer drops of essential oil because the skin of the face is much more delicate and requires only small amounts for effective treatment. Your choice of blends and carriers will depend on the skin type of the receiver (see table, below).

**SUGGESTED FACE AND DÉCOLLETAGE MASSAGE BLENDS**

Some of the carrier oils suggested here are deeply enriching and have been specially chosen to nourish the delicate skin of the face and décolletage area. If you do not have the carrier oil that is suggested for a particular blend, it is fine to use a substitute such as sweet almond oil. The blend you choose can be used to massage both the face and the décolletage area as one treatment.

| SKIN TYPE | DESCRIPTION | BLENDS |
|---|---|---|
| Dry skin | Fine textured, easily flushed by wind or cold | Rose 2 drops, Sandalwood 2 drops in 4tsp apricot kernel oil |
| Oily skin | Large pores, shiny appearance, slightly coarse in texture | Cypress 1 drop, Petitgrain 3 drops in 4tsp grapeseed oil |
| Acne-prone skin | Suffering outbreaks of inflammation and pimples | Manuka 2 drops, Lemon 2 drops in 4tsp jojoba oil |
| Combination skin | Dry on the cheeks, but oily over the forehead, nose and chin areas | Geranium 2 drops, Mandarin 2 drops in 4tsp camellia oil |
| Mature skin | More lined, with a tendency to look tired and undernourished | Rose 2 drops, Neroli 2 drops in 4tsp kukui nut oil |
| Sensitive skin | Prone to allergies especially to skincare products | Rose 2 drops, Yarrow 2 drops in 4tsp jojoba oil |
| Weather-damaged skin | More lined, perhaps with broken veins or a leathery appearance | Frankincense 2 drops, Neroli 2 drops in 4tsp kukui nut oil |

"Décolletage" is a French word which refers to the area from the neck down to just above the chest area. In Swedish massage it is common to massage the breast area itself, but while men usually do not find this problematic, many women feel uncomfortable. An acceptable alternative is to massage to the décolletage area as well as the face.

## STRUCTURE OF THE FACE AND DÉCOLLETAGE

The face is made up of a network of tiny muscles that attach to the bony skull underneath. These allow us to move, speak and show feelings or emotions through our facial expressions. On top of this layer of muscles sits the skin, which is much finer in texture in this area of the body than elsewhere and needs more nourishment. Exposure to the elements and forming habitual facial expressions can result in our skin becoming taut and tired-looking or showing fine lines. Massage restores good blood supply to the area and improves the skin's appearance. The décolletage consists of the skin overlying the collar bones, the upper chest area and the top of the breastbone.

## FACE AND DÉCOLLETAGE MASSAGE SAFETY CHECK

Before you start work assess the skin to be treated. If the person has allergies to face-care products, use the sensitive skin blend. If they have skin damage through overexposure to the sun or wind, use the damaged skin blend. If they have severe acne, don't work; if it affects only certain areas, work around them. If they have eczema or psoriasis, don't work and refer them to a skin specialist.

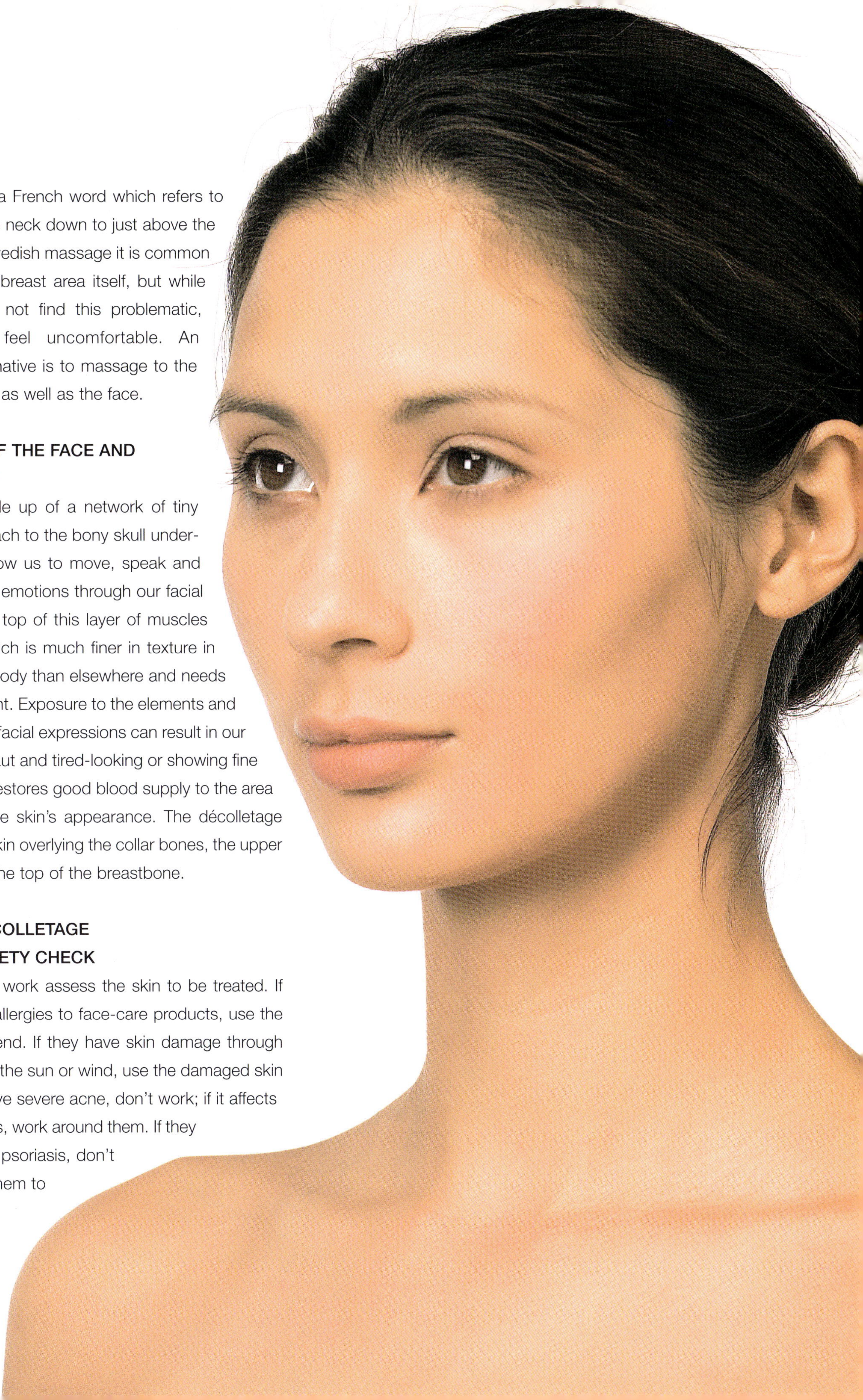

# FACE MASSAGE ROUTINE

To set up your treatment, invite the recipient to lie on their back on your futon mattress or foam pad with a pillow or folded towel under their knees and another under their head for extra support. Lay one towel horizontally over the upper body, and one lengthwise over the legs. Add a blanket over the whole body to keep it warm while you work. Fold the top towel down over the blanket to just above the breast area.

The receiver should remove glasses, contact lenses and any make-up before the treatment; for a pleasant start you can wipe their skin gently with a cotton wool pad soaked in lavender or rose flower water as a freshener. Kneel above the head to work. Make sure you have enough room to kneel comfortably with your back straight.

When you are performing this routine, let your movements be slow, gentle and deliberate. Face massage is extremely relaxing for the recipient, and very often they will fall asleep while you are working! You will need about 1tsp (5ml) of your chosen blend.

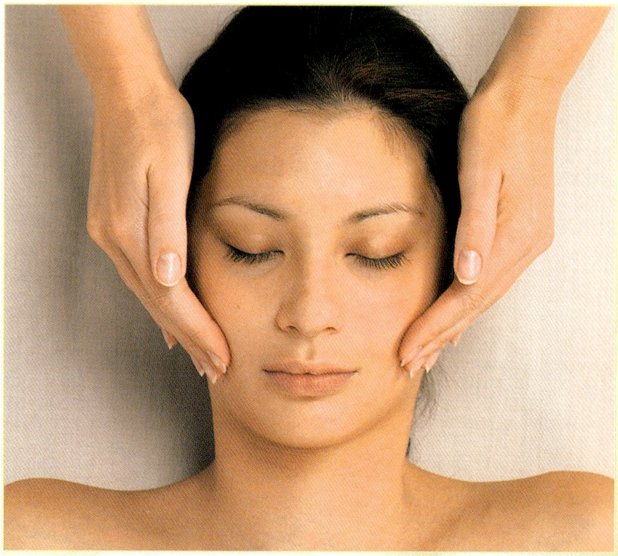

**1. Fingertip effleurage:** Starting with both hands together in the middle of the hairline, make tiny circles with your fingertips across the forehead, down both cheeks, over the top of the lips and around the chin, then sweep gently back over the cheeks and up to the forehead. Repeat this sequence three times.

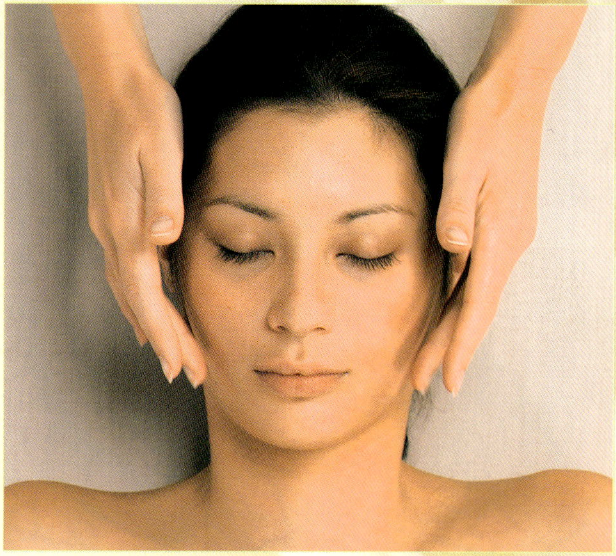

**4. Gentle fingertip tapping:** Using both hands tap very gently all over the face with your fingertips – it should feel almost like drops of water. Keep your movements extremely light and don't move into the eye area. This technique helps to stimulate the circulation.

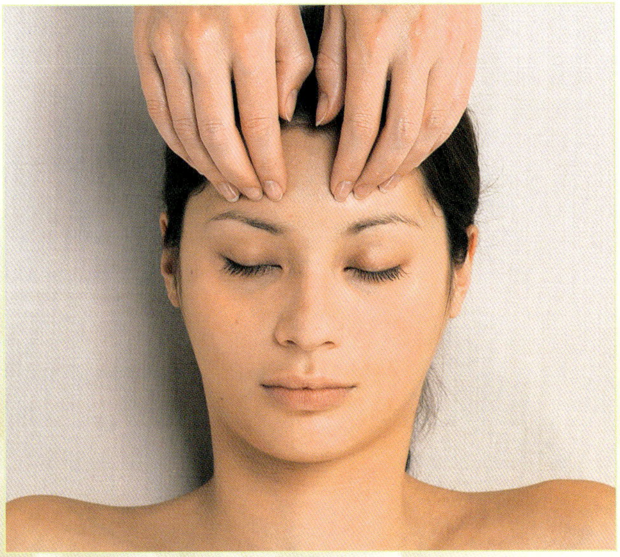

**2. Gentle fingertip pressures:** Again starting with both hands in the middle of the hairline, make lines of gentle pressures horizontally down the forehead to the eyebrows; then very gently all around the bony ridge of the eye socket. Do not go into the delicate eye area. Sweep up the nose to end, and then repeat this sequence twice.

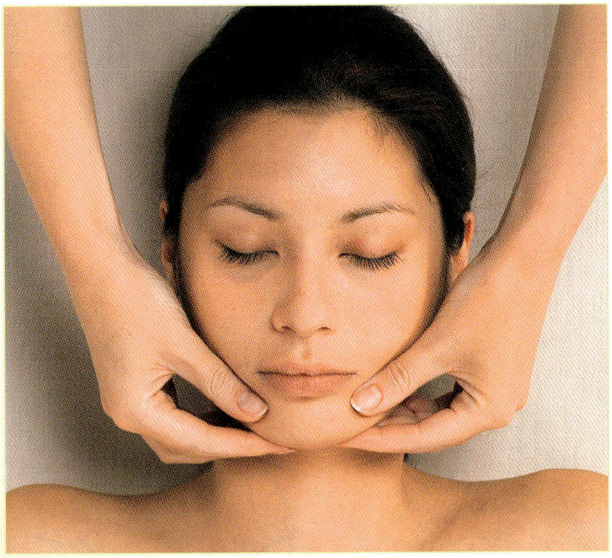

**3. Gentle fingertip kneading:** Bring both hands down to just under each ear, using your thumb and fingertips gently knead all the way round the chin until your hands meet in the middle. Then reverse the action and work back out to the sides. Repeat this sequence twice.

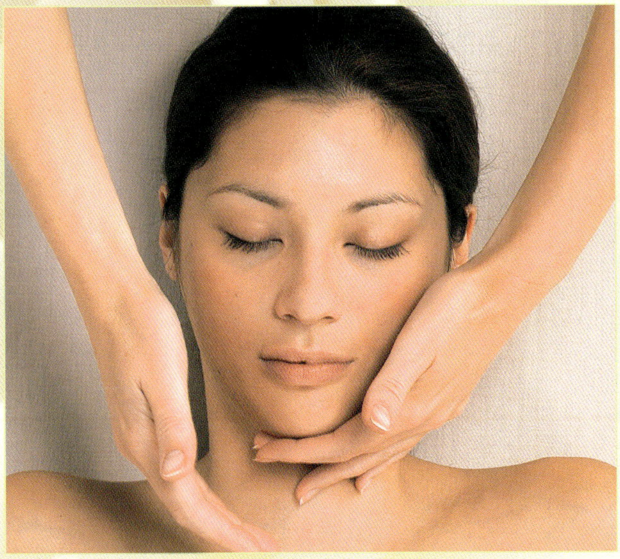

**5. Sweeping strokes:** With both hands make soft sweeping strokes upward, one hand after the other, first under the chin, then over the cheeks, the sides of the temples and up the forehead. Repeat this sequence twice, slowing down and getting lighter as you do it for the last time.

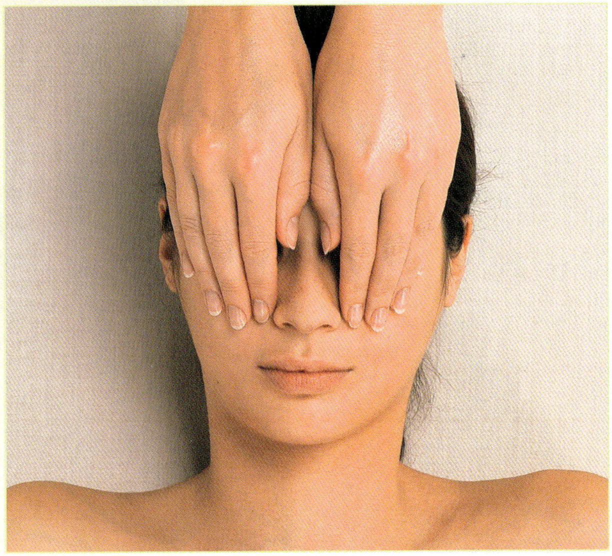

**6. Resting over the eyes:** To finish the routine, hold your hands just over the recipient's eyes, not actually touching them. They will still feel the warmth from your hands. This feels very relaxing to receive and also soothes the eyes themselves.

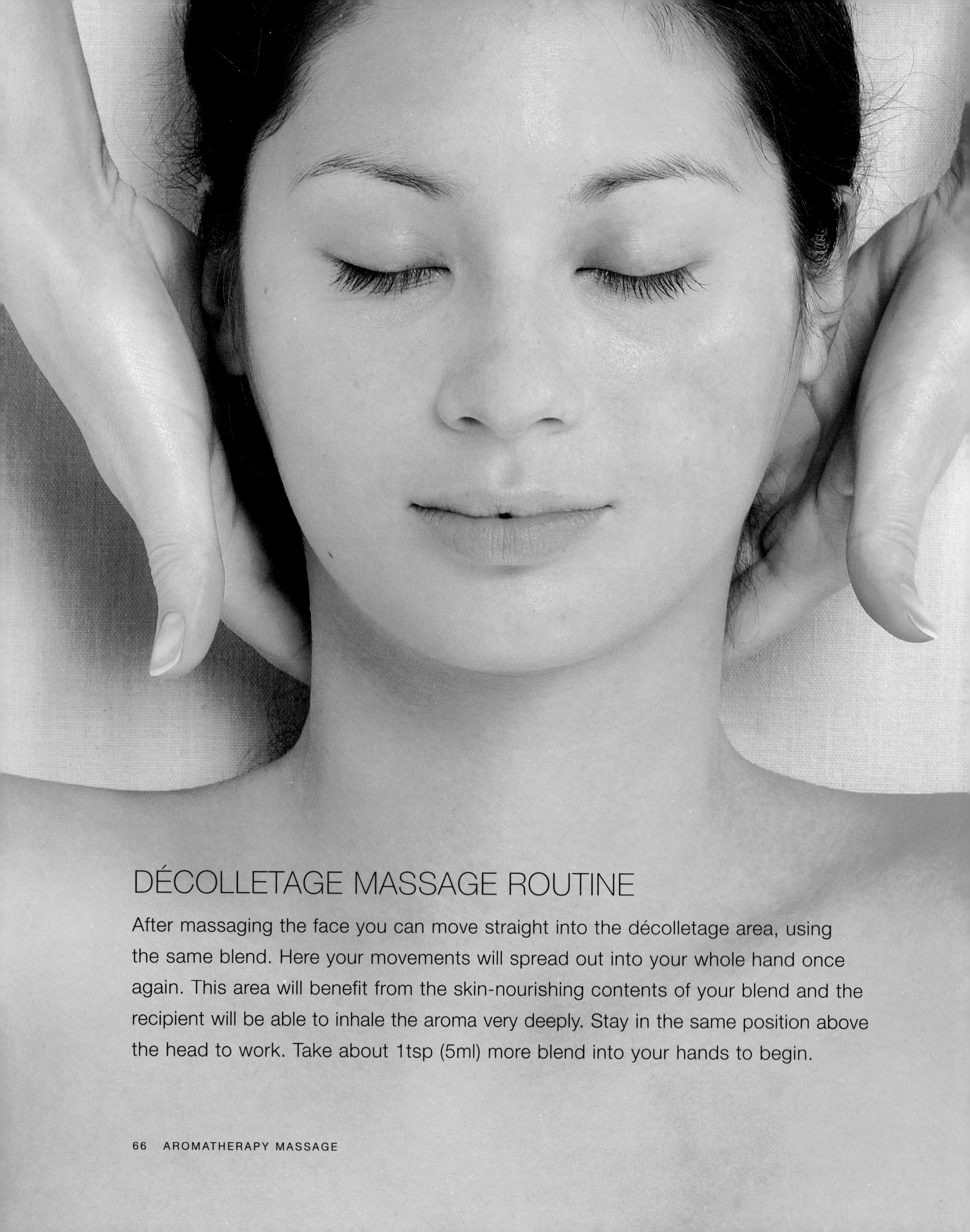

# DÉCOLLETAGE MASSAGE ROUTINE

After massaging the face you can move straight into the décolletage area, using the same blend. Here your movements will spread out into your whole hand once again. This area will benefit from the skin-nourishing contents of your blend and the recipient will be able to inhale the aroma very deeply. Stay in the same position above the head to work. Take about 1tsp (5ml) more blend into your hands to begin.

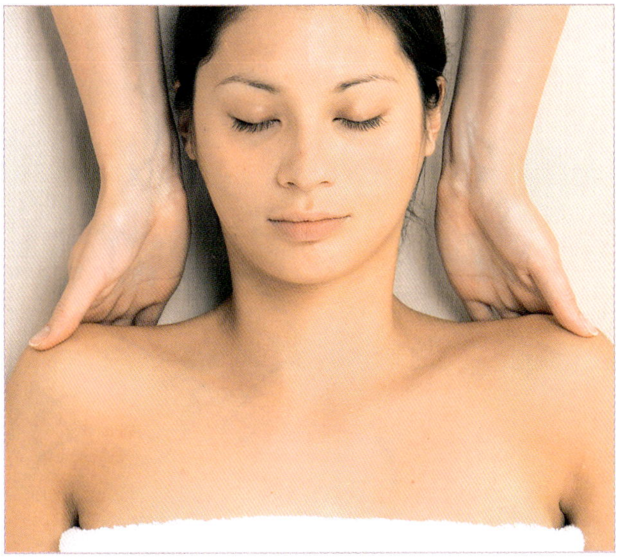

**1. Effleurage:** Starting with both hands under the top of the neck by the hairline, stroke down over both shoulders, then across and down to the middle of the décolletage area, then back across to the shoulders and up the neck again. Repeat this sequence four times, moving slowly and deliberately, with firm but not heavy pressure.

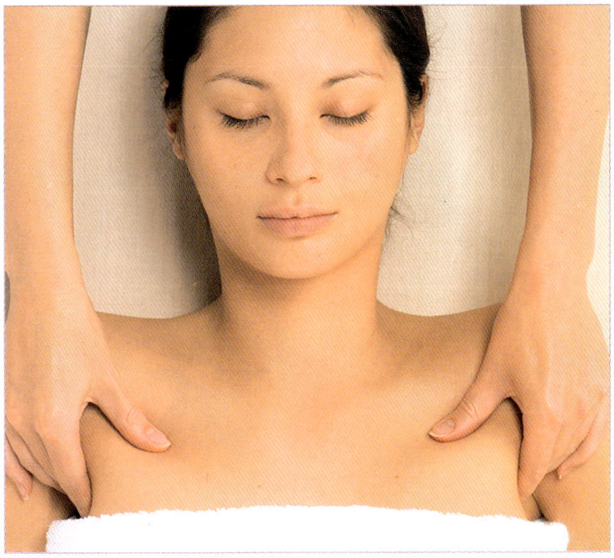

**2. Kneading the pectorals:** The large pectoral muscles across the chest often become tense just above the armpits, sometimes as a result of activities such as driving, lifting or typing; with one hand on each side, apply single-handed kneading into this area.

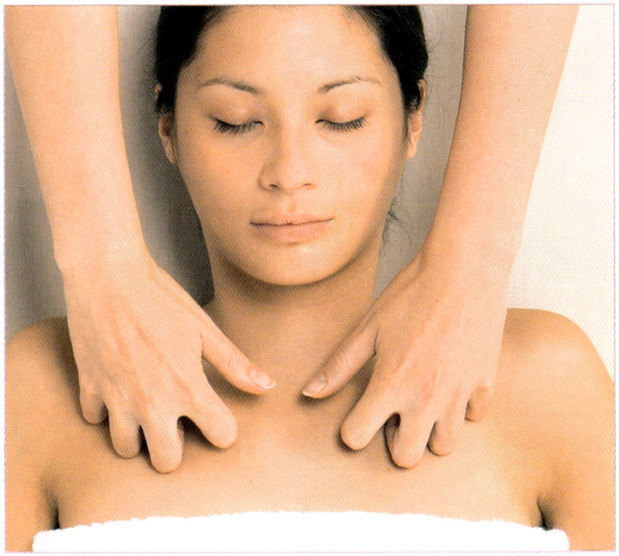

**3. Knuckling:** With your hands in loose fists, gently knuckle all over the décolletage area, checking with the recipient that the pressure is good; if you wish, you can also knuckle into the tops of the shoulders while you are working in this area.

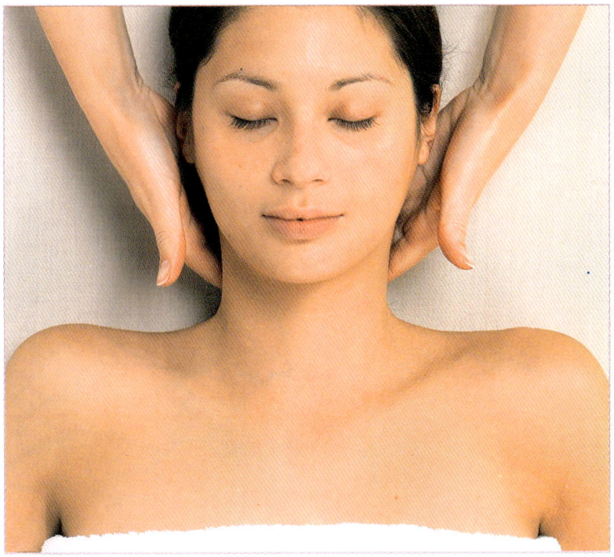

**4. Sweeping strokes:** To finish the routine, gently sweep your hands upward over the area, toward the chin, then up the sides of the shoulders, to finish with your hands gently holding under the neck as you began. Rest there for a moment or two to end.

# hand massage

The hands benefit greatly from massage. Working hard every day, our hands and are often exposed to harsh substances such as detergents. Massage eases stiffness and improves the circulation, and the aromatherapy blend improves skin texture.

### HAND MASSAGE SAFETY CHECK

Before you start work, examine the hands. Are there any injuries? If yes, don't massage. Does the person have arthritis in the hands? If severe, don't massage; if mild, work very gently. Are there any skin problems present, such as eczema? If yes, use the soothing blend, right.

### SETTING UP YOUR TREATMENT

Invite the receiver to sit opposite you. Place a towel over your lap and then hold their left hand on your right knee. Swap sides when you come to massage the other hand. You will need about 1tsp (5ml) of the blend for each hand, or more if the skin is very dry.

**SUGGESTED HAND MASSAGE BLENDS**

Make up any of the following blends in a carrier of 4tsp (20ml) sweet almond oil, which is an excellent hand-conditioner.

| BENEFITS | BLENDS |
|---|---|
| Skin-soothing | Lavender 6 drops, Yarrow 2 drops, Geranium 2 drops |
| Circulation-warming | Ginger 2 drops, Cardamom 4 drops, Sweet orange 4 drops |
| Super-treatment | Neroli 4 drops, Rose 2 drops, Frankincense 4 drops |

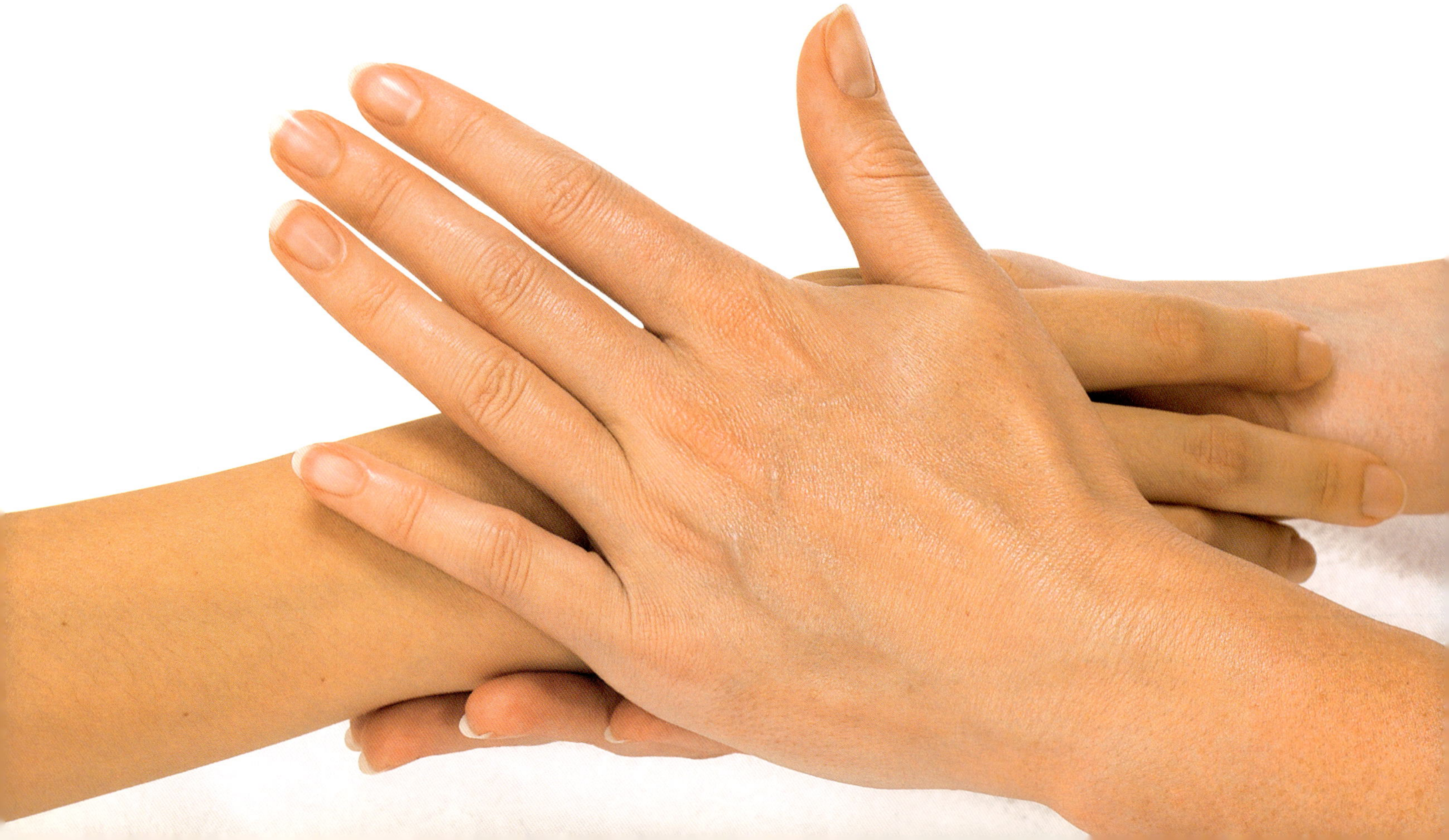

# HAND MASSAGE ROUTINE

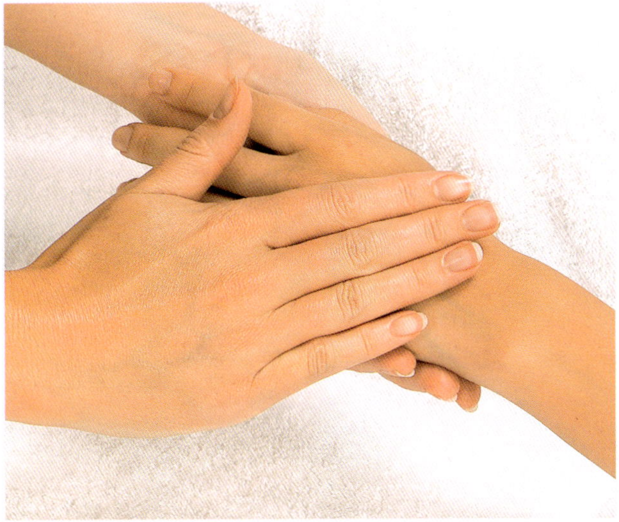

**1. Effleurage:** Support the receiver's left hand with your left hand holding it palm down on your knee. With your right hand, stroke upward from their fingertips toward their wrist, easing off pressure as you glide back to the fingertips. Repeat several times, particularly if the hand is cold.

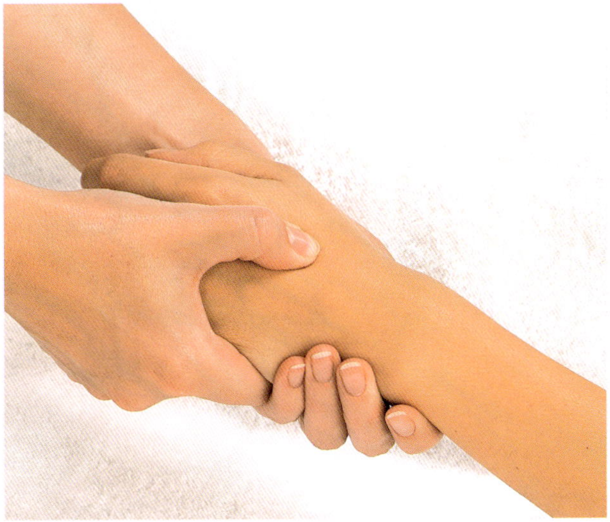

**2. Thumb pressures on upper surface:** With their hand still supported palm down on your knee, use your thumb to trace the lines of pressure between the bones, up toward the wrist. You should be able to fee four such lines covering the hand; Repeat this sequence three times.

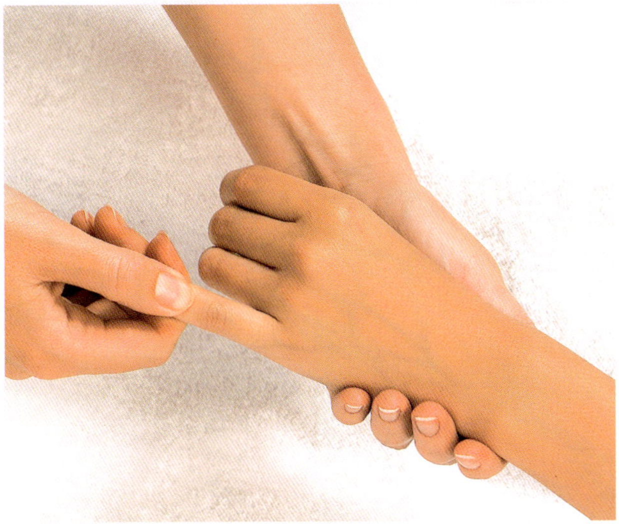

**3. Kneading the fingers:** Still supporting the hand, use your other hand to carefully squeeze and knead each of the fingers and the thumb in turn, working all the way from the nails down to where the digits join the palm. Take your time over this, it feels very relaxing to receive.

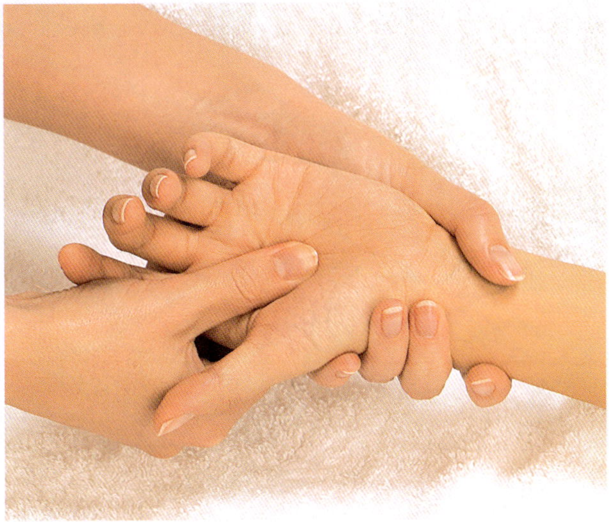

**4. Circle pressures in the palm:** Turn the hand palm up and continue to support it. Using your thumb, make firm circular pressures over the surface of the palm, in a slow relaxed rhythm. To finish, turn the hand palm down again and repeat step 1. Repeat the routine on the right hand.

# foot massage

It is said that the feet will carry you to the moon and back in a lifetime, and, mostly, they get precious little attention. Some people really dislike their feet, which is a pity because they are quite miraculous structures that are sensitive to the environment, and exquisitely formed and balanced so that we can walk upright. A good foot massage is bliss at the end of a long day and can help to relax the entire body.

### FOOT MASSAGE SAFETY CHECK

Before you start work, examine the feet. Are there any infections present, such as verrucae or athlete's foot? If yes, don't massage. Are there any areas of badly damaged skin, such as on the heels? If yes, use the skin-healing blend, right. Are there any injuries to the feet, such as sprains or broken bones? If yes, don't massage.

### SETTING UP YOUR TREATMENT

The recipient should lie on the futon or foam mattress on their back, covered with a blanket, and with their feet wrapped in a towel. Ideally, the feet should be washed beforehand, or use a wet wipe to refresh them. Sit or kneel at the feet to work. Unwrap one foot at a time to work and cover it afterward.

**SUGGESTED FOOT MASSAGE BLENDS**

Make up any of the following blends in 4tsp (20ml) jojoba oil, which is a good skin-healing carrier.

| BENEFITS | BLENDS |
|---|---|
| Warming and circulation-stimulating | Black pepper 4 drops, Nutmeg 2 drops, Lavendin 4 drops |
| Refreshing and cooling | Peppermint 4 drops, Lemon 4 drops, Eucalyptus 2 drops |
| Skin-healing | German chamomile 2 drops, Myrrh 4 drops, Frankincense 4 drops |

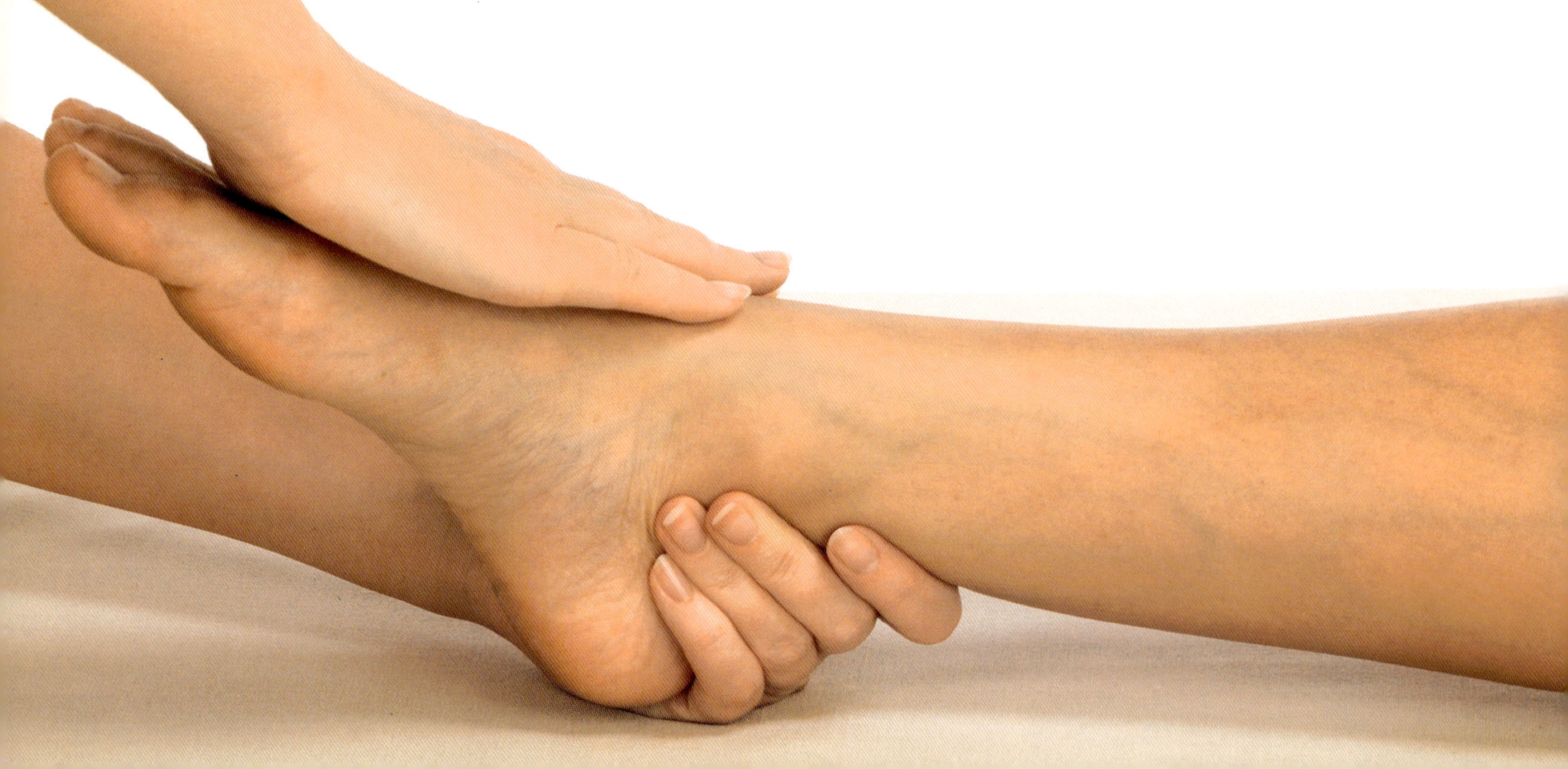

# FOOT MASSAGE ROUTINE

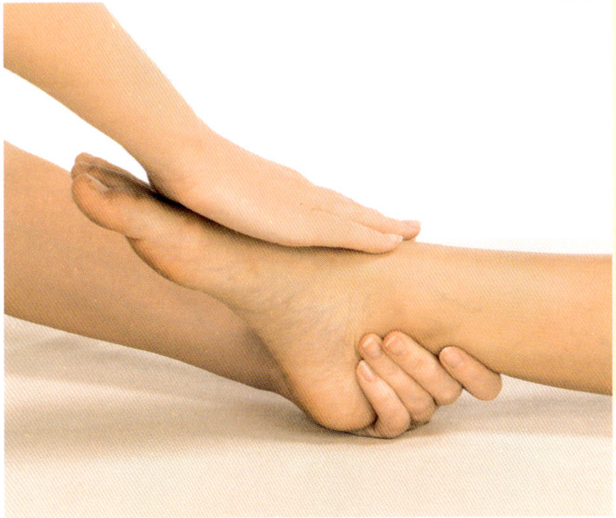

1. **Effleurage:** Start with the right foot, supporting it under the ankle with your left hand. With your right hand stroke from the toes over the upper surface of the foot toward the ankle, then glide back. Pressure should be firm upward and light downward. Repeat several times.

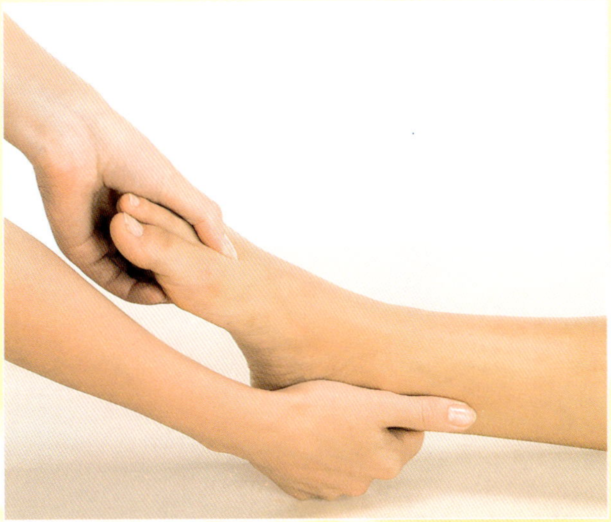

2. **Thumb pressures on upper surface:** Still supporting the foot, trace the four lines of pressure from the creases between the toes down toward the ankle, starting by the little toe and working across toward the big toe. This may feel tender so take care with the pressure you apply.

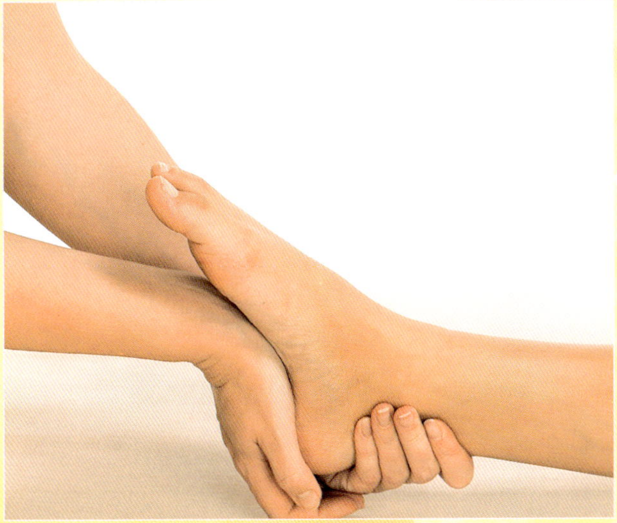

3. **Heel of hand under arch:** Supporting the ankle with your left hand, use the soft pad at the base of your right wrist to slowly and firmly rub up and down the sole and arch of the foot. Feel the way the foot moves as you do this – it really stretches it out and eases stiffness.

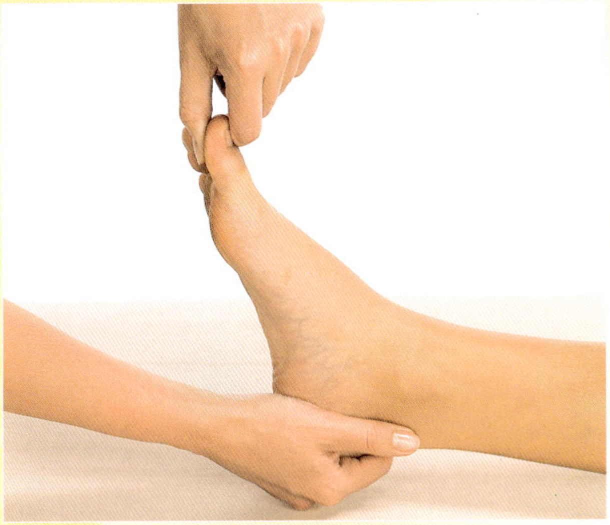

4. **Kneading the toes:** Support the foot under the ankle with your other hand. Carefully and gently stretch and massage each of the toes in turn, rubbing the blend in well. To finish your foot massage, repeat step 1. Now repeat the routine on the left foot.

# abdomen massage

This is an area that carries a lot of physical and emotional tension. It is important to work sensitively so that your touch feels nurturing and reassuring.

### ABDOMEN MASSAGE SAFETY CHECK

Before you start, check the following. Is the intended recipient pregnant? If yes, check their midwife is happy for massage to be given, and work gently with a diluted blend (see pp.26–27). Are there any digestive problems? If severe, don't massage; if mild to moderate, work gently. If there is period pain, massage very gently.

### SETTING UP YOUR TREATMENT

Invite the receiver to lie on their back on the futon or mattress. Place a towel over their chest and another over their legs, leaving the abdomen unwrapped. Kneel on their right side facing across the abdomen.

**SUGGESTED ABDOMEN MASSAGE BLENDS**

Make up any of the following blends in a carrier of 4tsp (20ml) sweet almond oil, for daytime or evening massage.

| BENEFITS | BLENDS |
|---|---|
| Soothing and relaxing | Lavender 2 drops, Roman chamomile 4 drops, Neroli 4 drops |
| Antispasmodic | Peppermint 4 drops, Sweet marjoram 4 drops, Ginger 2 drops |
| Warming and digestive tonic | Turmeric 2 drops, Cardamom 4 drops, Sweet orange 4 drops |

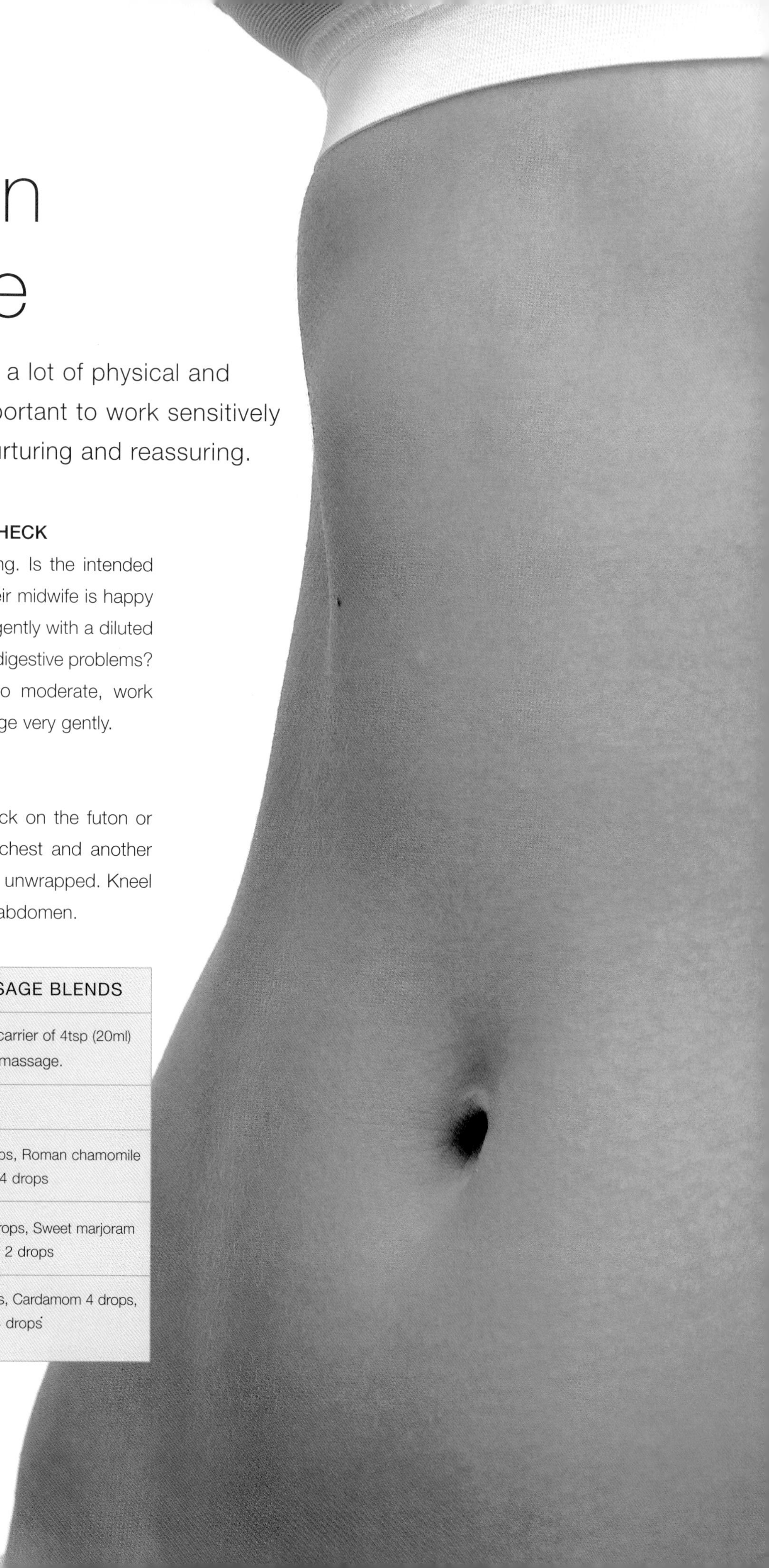

# ABDOMEN MASSAGE ROUTINE

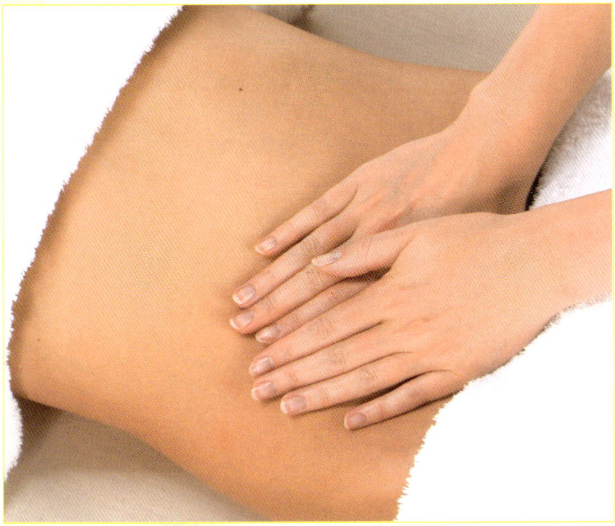

**1. Circle effleurage:** Using both hands next to each other, stroke the abdomen from the right hip, up over the ribs, down to the left hip and across the lower stomach. Repeat several times. Do this slowly and use light pressure.

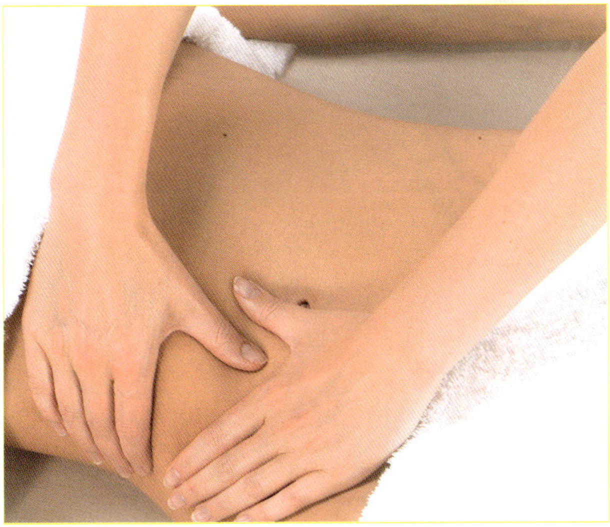

**2. Kneading:** Using both hands, pick up and knead the flesh on the left side of the abdomen, slowly and carefully, then do the same on the right side. Make sure that the pressure is firm; if it is too light your touch may tickle.

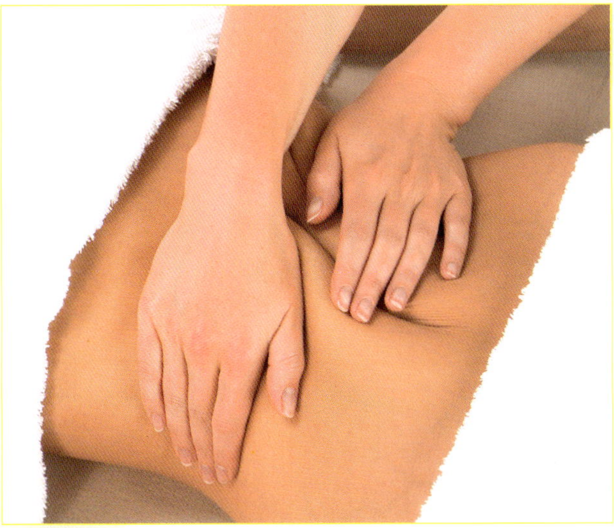

**3. Criss-cross effleurage:** Place one hand on the far side of the abdomen and one on the nearest side to you. Stroke across the area so that your hands criss-cross each other alternately. Keep the rhythm slow and soothing.

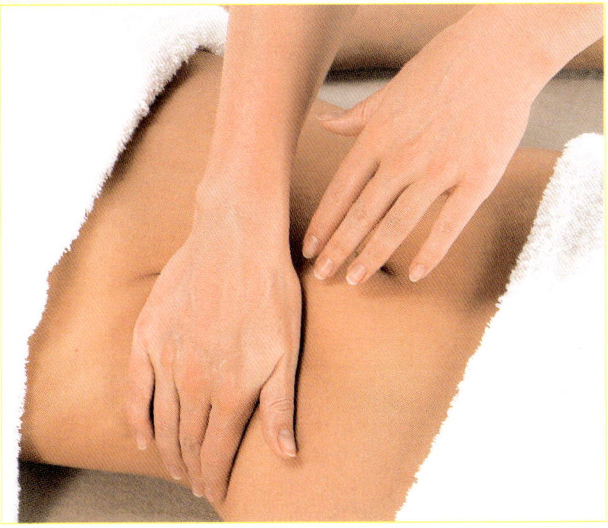

**4. Side stroking:** With both hands on the far side of the abdomen, let one hand follow the other in a gentle alternate stroke up over the area; then bring your hands to the near side, and push across, again using the hands one after the other. To finish the massage, repeat step 1.

# arm massage

The arms respond well to massage because they are often very tired as a result of all the tasks they have to do each day. The muscles are easy to find although they are fairly small, so your movements often need only one hand rather than two.

### ARM MASSAGE SAFETY CHECK

Before you start any work, ask the intended recipient a few questions to assess whether or not to proceed. Are there any injuries to the arms such as muscular pulls or broken bones? If yes, don't work. Are there any repetitive strain problems in any areas, or persistent aches and pains? If yes, work gently and carefully over these areas.

### SETTING UP YOUR TREATMENT

Invite the person to lie on their back on the futon or mattress, on top of a clean sheet. Place a flat pillow or folded towel under their head. Fold a towel lengthways and place it under the arm on which you are working, to raise it slightly. Cover the rest of the body to keep the person warm. Make up your blend, then kneel by their hip on the side of the arm you are treating.

**SUGGESTED ARM MASSAGE BLENDS**

Make up any of the following blends in a carrier of 4tsp (20ml) jojoba oil, an excellent all-round skin-conditioner.

| BENEFITS | BLENDS |
|---|---|
| Pain-relieving | German chamomile 2 drops, Lavender 6 drops, Vetiver 2 drops |
| Circulation-boosting | Rosemary 4 drops, Black pepper 4 drops, Lemongrass 2 drops |
| Muscle-warming | Sweet marjoram 4 drops, Coriander seed 4 drops, May chang 2 drops |

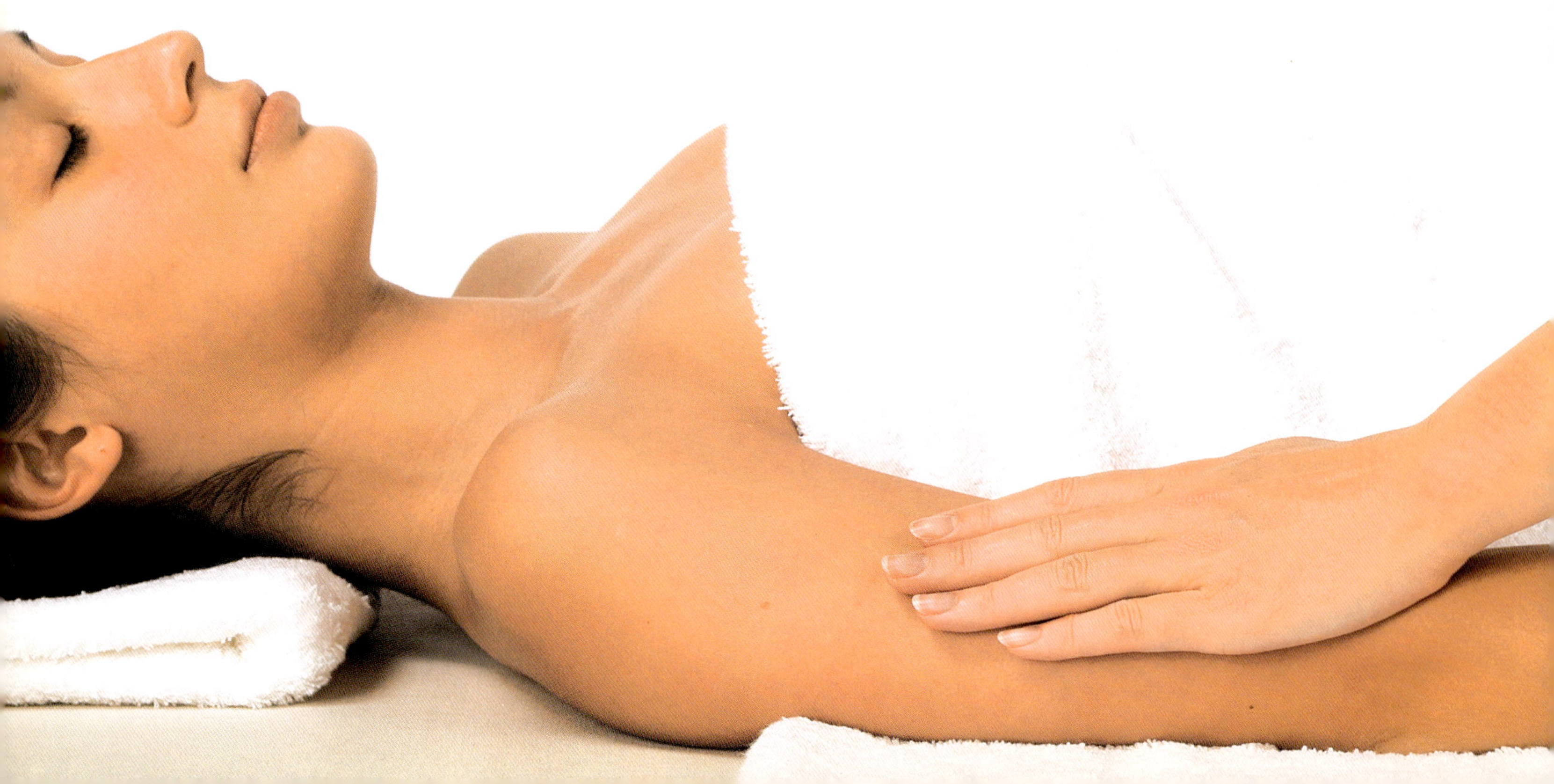

# ARM MASSAGE ROUTINE

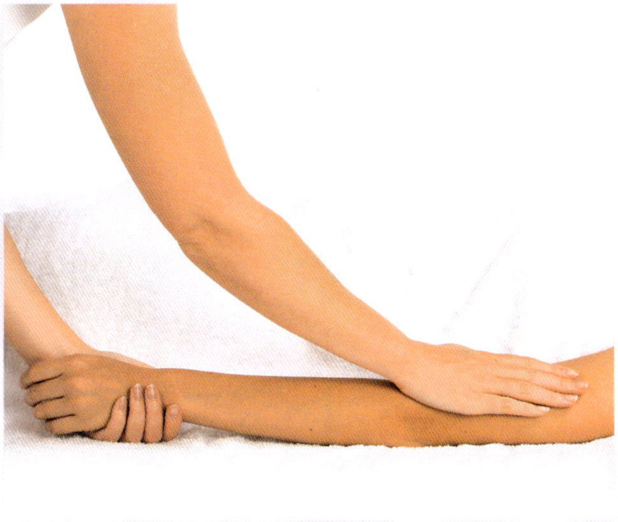

1. **Effleurage:** Hold the wrist lightly with one of your hands to support it. With the other hand stroke all the way up the arm from the fingertips to the shoulders, and back down again. The pressure should be firm as you go up, and light as you come down. Repeat this several times.

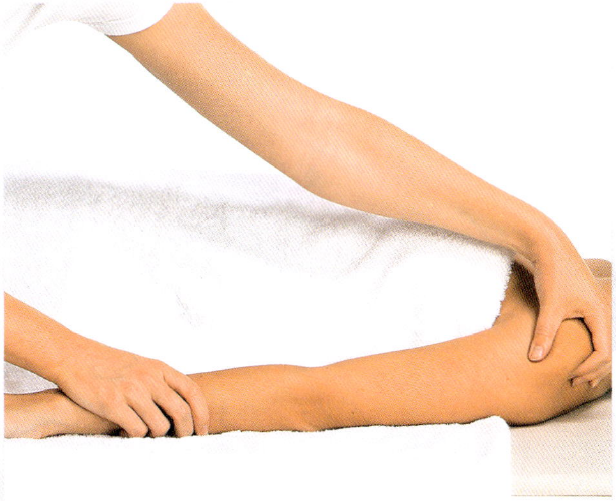

2. **Kneading (upper arm):** Still supporting the arm with one hand, use your other hand to knead across the shoulder area, down the sides of the arm and into the muscles as far as the elbow crease. Keep working until the area feels warm and supple; check that the pressure feels good.

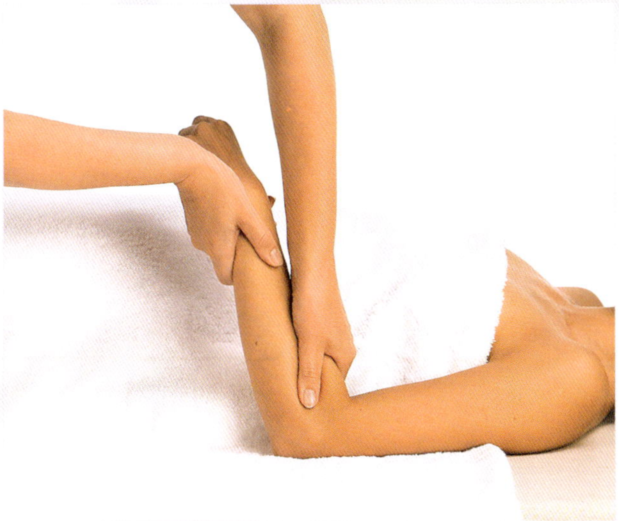

3. **Draining (lower arm):** Now bend the arm at the elbow and hold the wrist securely with one of your hands while you use your other hand to stroke slowly and firmly down from the wrist to the elbow crease and back. The pressure should be firm as you go down and light as you glide back.

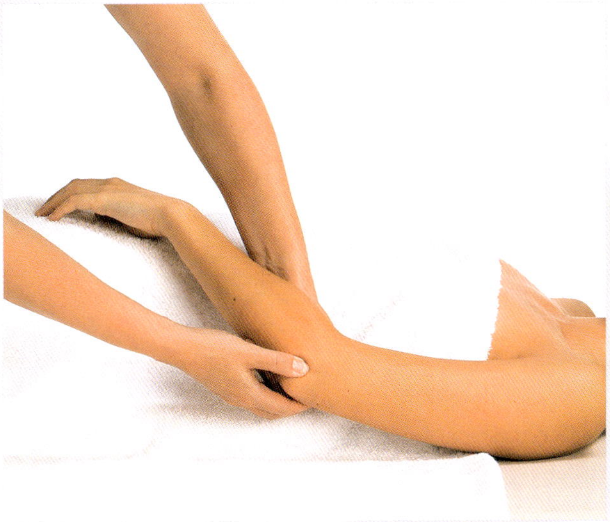

4. **Fingertip massage (elbow):** Slide both of your hands under the elbow and massage gently all around that area with your fingertips making little circular movements. To finish the treatment, repeat step 1. Now repeat the routine on the other arm.

# leg massage

Working on the legs can be more or less challenging depending on the size of the person you are treating. If they have larger muscles and heavier legs you will find it a more physically demanding massage. However, it is always relaxing to receive.

## LEG MASSAGE SAFETY CHECK

Before you start any work, ask the intended recipient a few questions to assess whether or not to proceed. Do they have any severe muscular problems in the legs? yes, don't massage. Do they have arthritis in any joints? If yes and severe, don't massage; if mild, work gently. Do they have varicose veins? If severe, don't massage; if mild to moderate, massage only above and below the area, with effleurage and no cupping movements.

## SETTING UP YOUR TREATMENT

Invite the person to lie on their back on the futon or mattress, on top of a clean sheet. Cover the top of their body and lay a towel lengthways over the legs, unwrapping one at a time to work. Kneel by the ankle of the leg you are massaging.

**SUGGESTED LEG MASSAGE BLENDS**

Make up any of the following blends in a carrier of 4tsp (20ml) jojoba oil, which will nourish the skin deeply.

| BENEFITS | BLENDS |
|---|---|
| Warming and stimulating | Peppermint 2 drops, Rosemary 4 drops, Nutmeg 4 drops |
| Soothing and pain-relieving | Vetiver 2 drops, Lavender 4 drops, Carrot seed 4 drops |
| Detoxifying and cleansing | Juniper 2 drops, Grapefruit 4 drops, Fennel 4 drops |

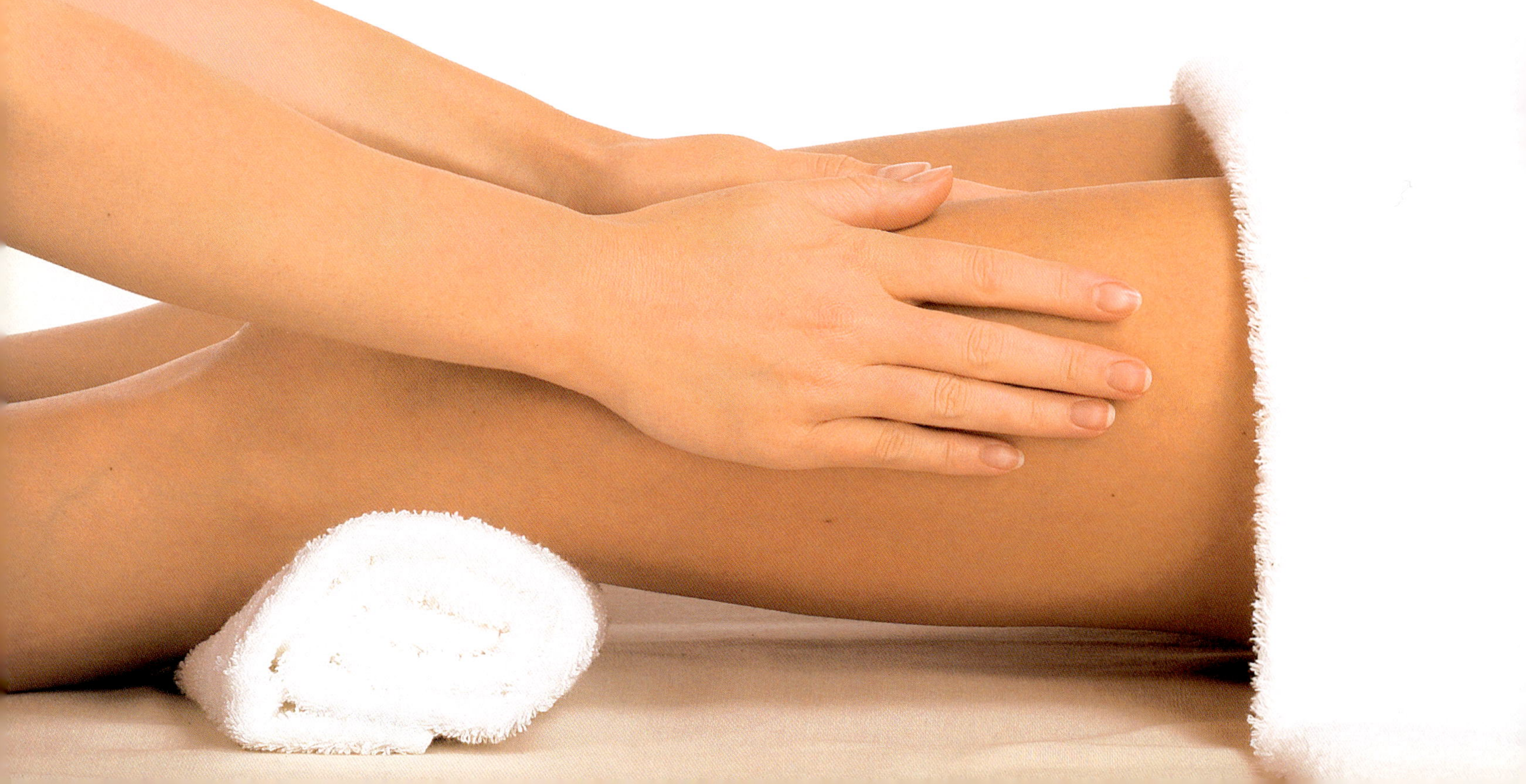

# LEG MASSAGE ROUTINE

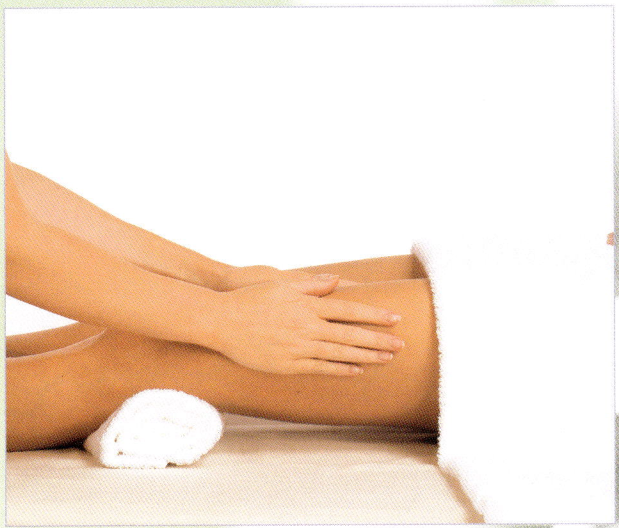

**1. Effleurage:** Place both hands just above the ankle and stroke all the way up toward the top of the leg, then glide back. Rock forward onto your knees to reach up and try to keep your back straight. Pressure should be firm as you go up and light as you glide down. Repeat several times.

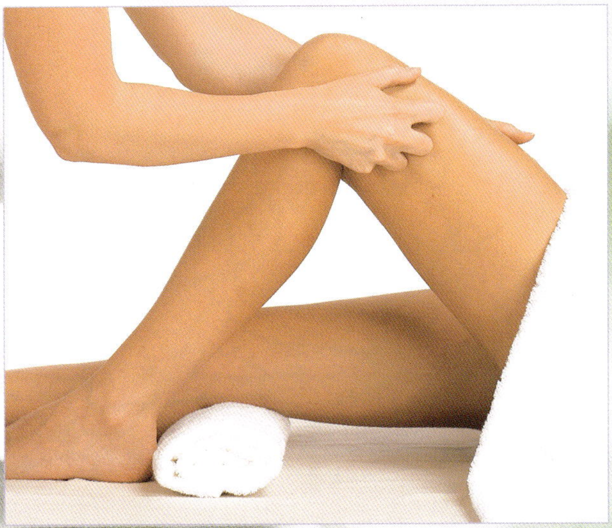

**2. Knuckling the thigh area:** Ask the person receiving the massage to bend their leg at the knee. Kneel beside it and knuckle all over the back of the thigh, and then over the top of the thigh. Check that the pressure you are applying at a comfortable level.

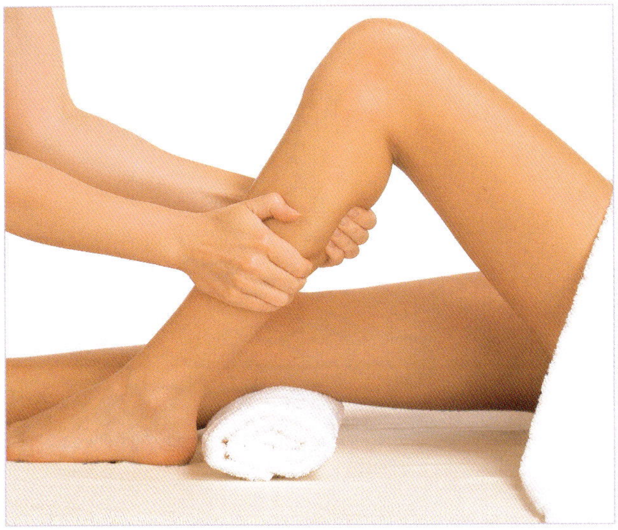

**3. Kneading the calf area:** Keep the leg bent at the knee, and adjust your position slightly so it is comfortable for you to use both hands to knead the muscles at the back of the calf. Squeeze them gently to ease out any stiffness.

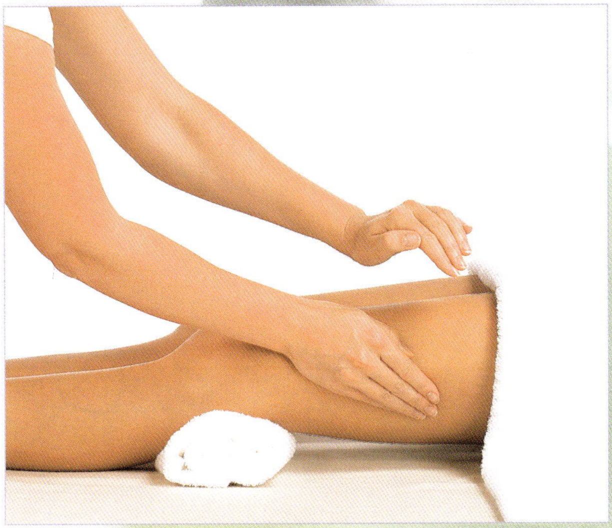

**4. Cupping the leg:** Lay the leg flat and tap lightly over the whole surface with loosely cupped hands to stimulate the circulation. Don't strike the skin too hard; cupping is brisk and leaves the leg tingling. To end, repeat step 1, then cover this leg and repeat the routine on the other one.

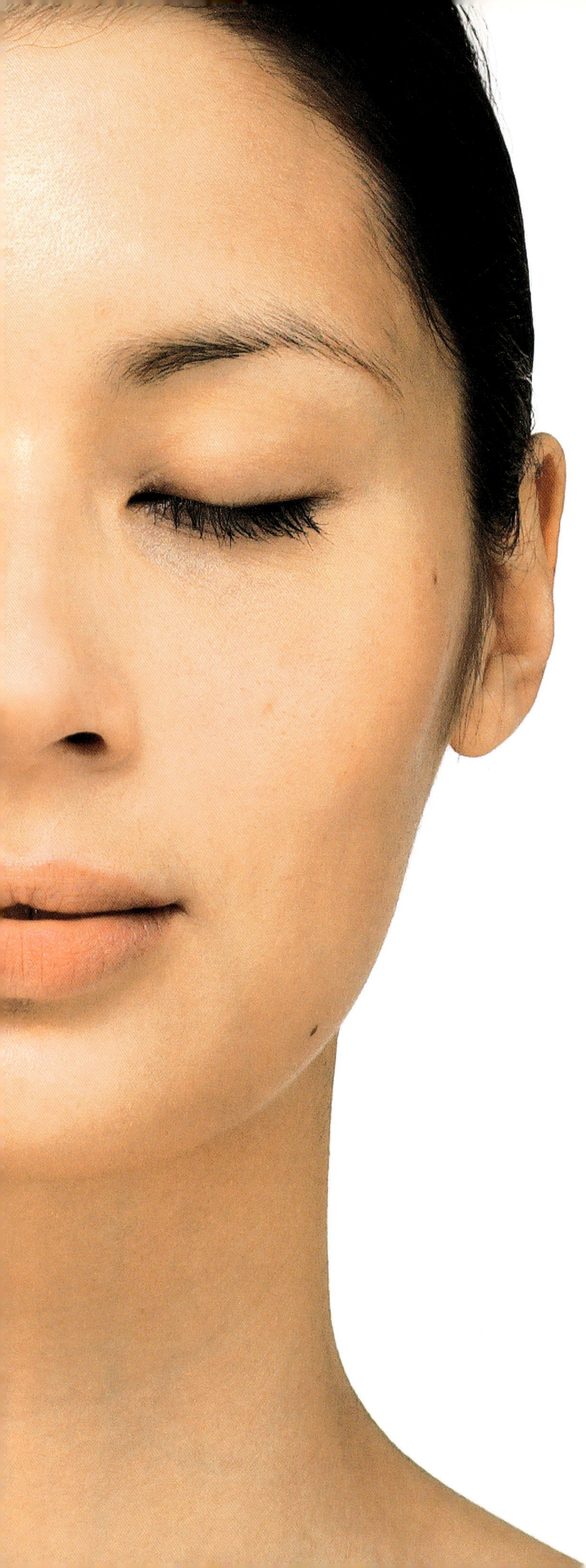

# self-massage of the face

Giving your own face an aromatherapy massage is a lovely treat – it nourishes the skin and makes you feel good. Specialist carrier oils such as apricot kernel or jojoba work best. All the blends suggested below are good for evening massage – the aromas relax you and will help you to sleep.

## FLORAL WATERS

These are pure aromatic waters, such as lavender, rose or neroli, which are the valuable by-products of essential oil distillation (see p.19). They make wonderful, gentle skin-toners, used after cleansing to remove excess product, and they refresh the skin before the massage treatment.

## AROMATHERAPY FACE-CARE ROUTINE

After removing make-up with your normal cleanser, try these simple steps:

- Dry/mature skin – *Tone:* use pure neroli water on a cotton wool pad to lightly refresh the skin; *face treatment massage oil:* 2tsp (10ml) jojoba with 2 drops Rose and 2 drops Neroli
- Oily/combination skin – *Tone:* use pure lavender water to deeply cleanse and gently tighten the pores; *face treatment massage oil:* 2tsp (10ml) jojoba with 2 drops Geranium and 2 drops Mandarin.
- Sensitive/delicate skin – *Tone:* use pure rose water to soothe and calm the skin; *face treatment massage oil:* 2tsp (10ml) apricot kernel with 1 drop Rose and 1 drop Rosewood.

# SELF-MASSAGE OF THE FACE ROUTINE

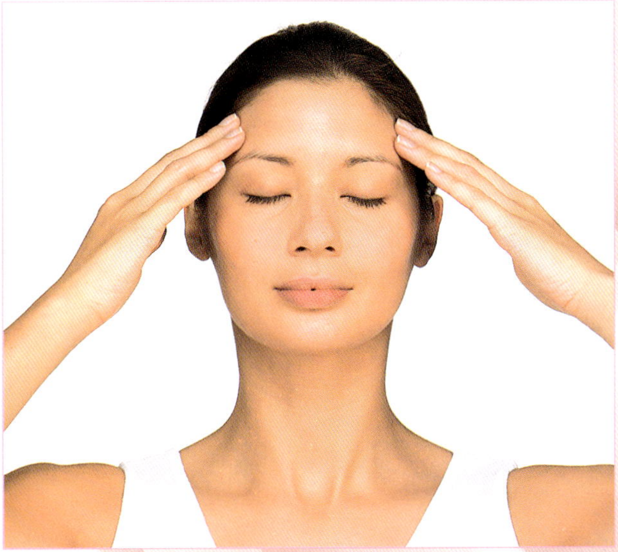

**1. Effleurage:** Put half a teaspoon (2.5ml) of blend on your hands and spread it to your fingertips. Stroke it over your forehead, down over your nose and cheeks, above your lips and over your chin. Repeat three times.

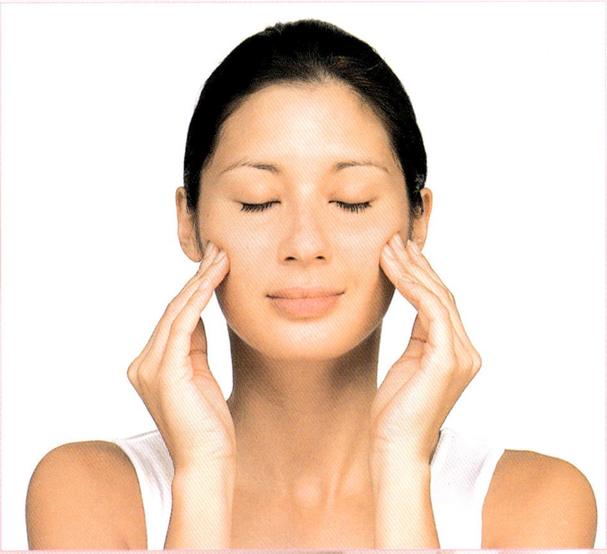

**2. Fingertip circles:** Using your fingertips and starting in the middle of your forehead, make tiny circular movements out to your temples, down your cheeks, across the top of your lips and over your chin. Repeat three times.

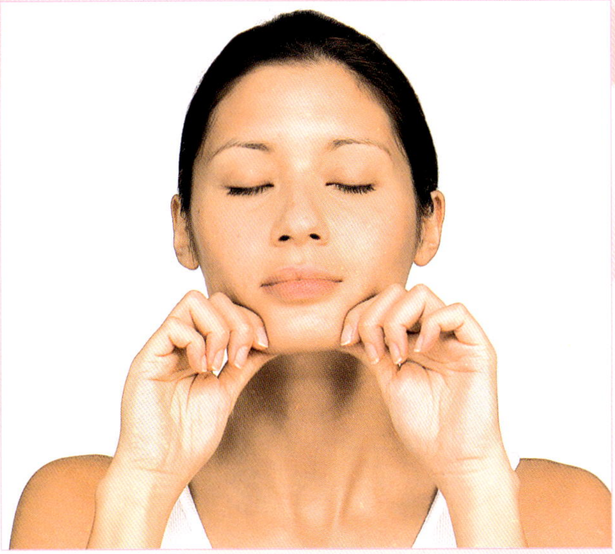

**3. Kneading the chin:** Using your fingertips and thumb, gently knead all along your chin, from just under your mouth out toward your ears and back again to really ease out your jaw. Repeat three times.

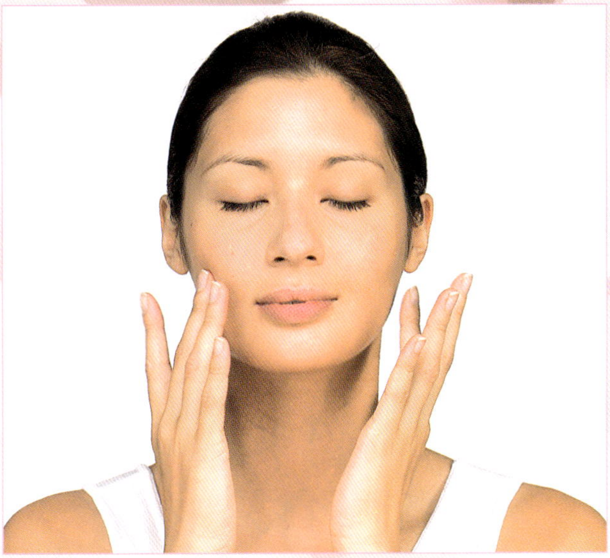

**4. Finger tapping:** Using the pads of your fingers, gently tap all over your face for a few moments to stimulate the circulation. This movement needs to be very light and soft, like drops of water. Finish by repeating step 1.

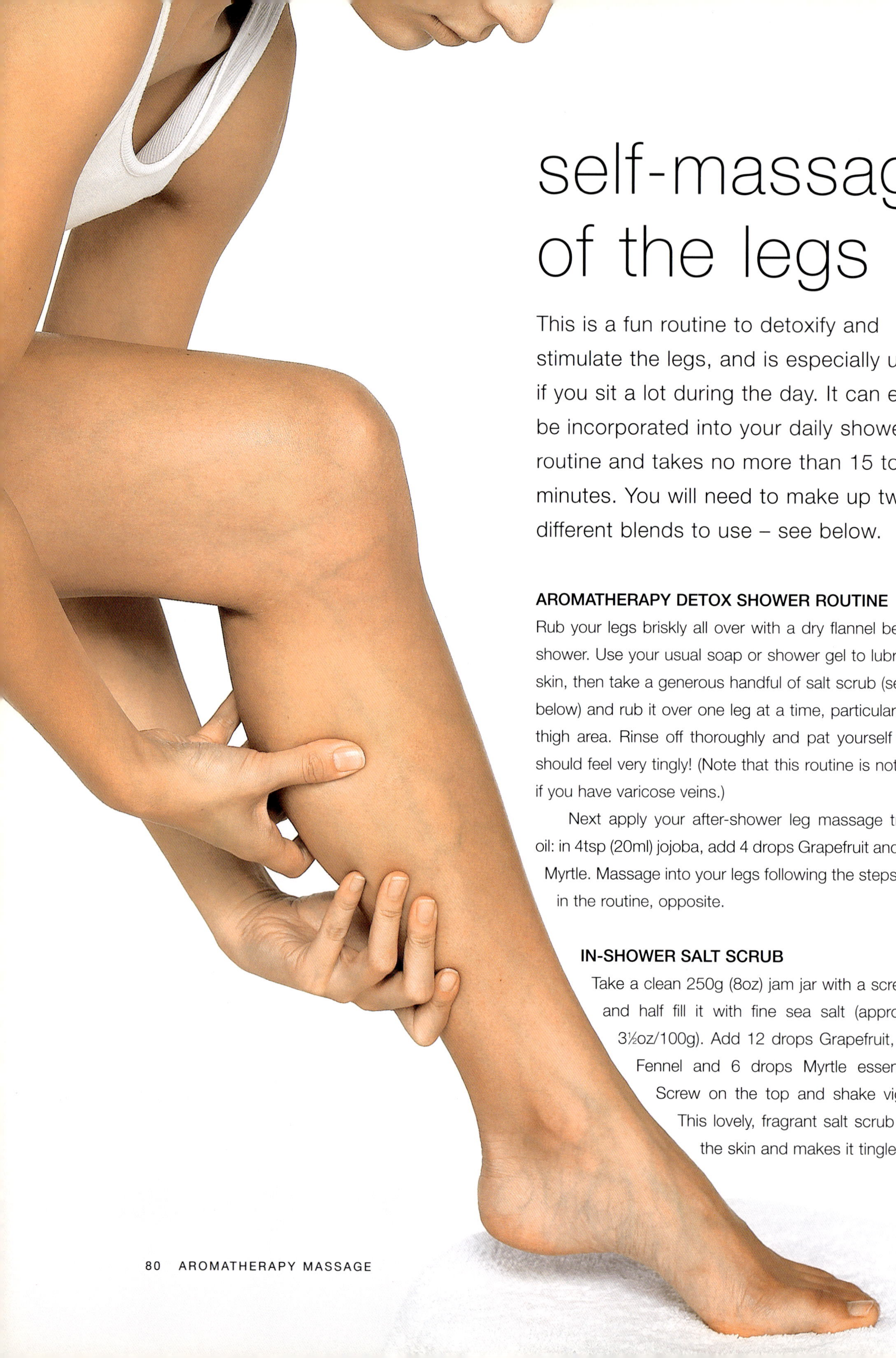

# self-massage of the legs

This is a fun routine to detoxify and stimulate the legs, and is especially useful if you sit a lot during the day. It can easily be incorporated into your daily shower routine and takes no more than 15 to 20 minutes. You will need to make up two different blends to use – see below.

## AROMATHERAPY DETOX SHOWER ROUTINE

Rub your legs briskly all over with a dry flannel before you shower. Use your usual soap or shower gel to lubricate the skin, then take a generous handful of salt scrub (see recipe below) and rub it over one leg at a time, particularly on the thigh area. Rinse off thoroughly and pat yourself dry. You should feel very tingly! (Note that this routine is not advised if you have varicose veins.)

Next apply your after-shower leg massage treatment oil: in 4tsp (20ml) jojoba, add 4 drops Grapefruit and 6 drops Myrtle. Massage into your legs following the steps outlined in the routine, opposite.

## IN-SHOWER SALT SCRUB

Take a clean 250g (8oz) jam jar with a screwtop lid and half fill it with fine sea salt (approximately 3½oz/100g). Add 12 drops Grapefruit, 6 drops Fennel and 6 drops Myrtle essential oils. Screw on the top and shake vigorously. This lovely, fragrant salt scrub enlivens the skin and makes it tingle.

# SELF-MASSAGE OF THE LEGS ROUTINE

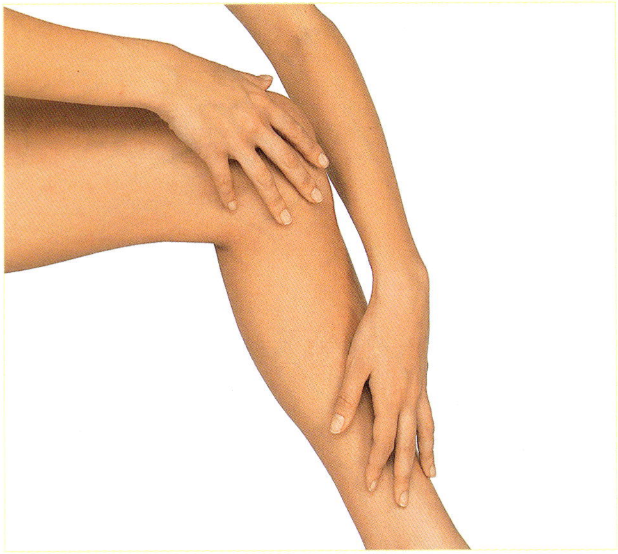

1. **Effleurage:** Take 1tsp (5ml) of your blend in your hands and rub them together gently. Stroke down your right leg so that the whole surface is well-covered. Really work it in well – the skin will absorb the jojoba base quickly.

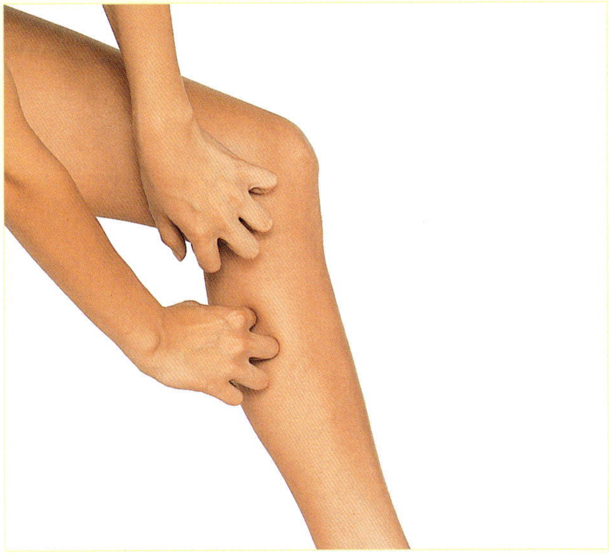

2. **Knuckling:** Using both hands make lightly clenched fists and gently work your knuckles down the whole leg, from the thigh to the ankle.

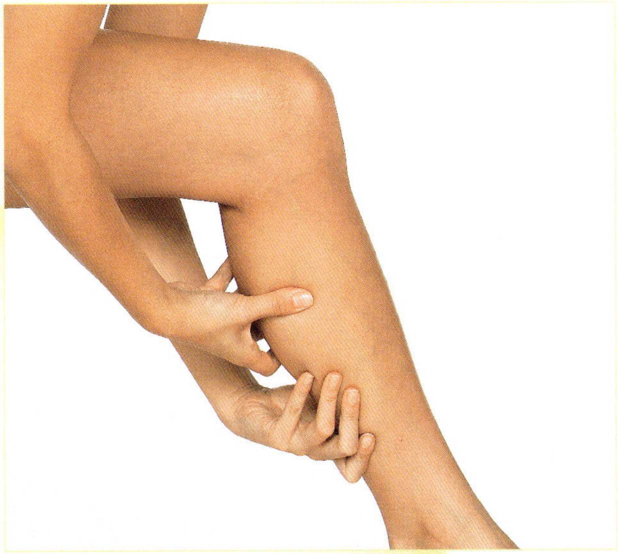

3. **Kneading:** Use one hand on each side of the leg and knead the muscles all the way down from the sides of the thighs to the calves. Now do the movement in reverse, kneading all the way back up again.

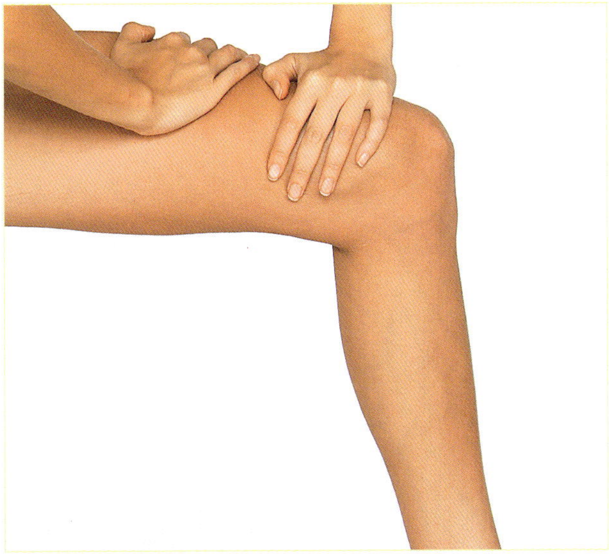

4. **Criss-crossing:** Place your hands on either side of the top of your thigh and stroke them across to the opposite sides in a criss-cross pattern. Go all down your leg and back up again. Nowdo the routine on your left leg.

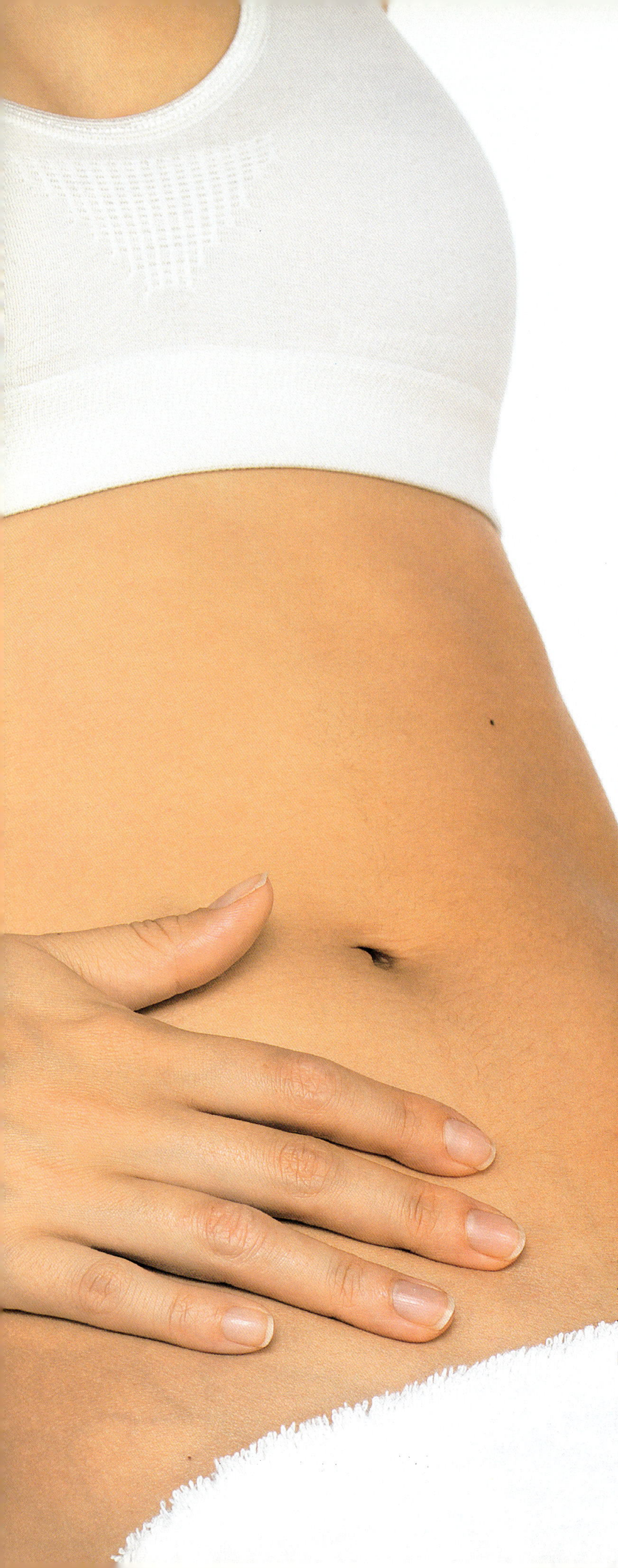

# self-massage of the abdomen

The abdomen holds tension and can experience cramps from stomach troubles or menstrual pain. Self-massage is extremely soothing because it helps you to relax, which in itself relieves discomfort. The essential oils used here ease muscular aches and cramps, as well as warming and relieving the area. Sit in a comfortable chair to give yourself this massage.

## SUGGESTED ABDOMEN SELF-MASSAGE BLENDS

If you are pregnant, only use half the number of drops of essential oils stated below in 4tsp (20ml) of sweet almond carrier oil.

- **Menstrual cramps** – Clary sage 4 drops, Sweet marjoram 4 drops and Ginger 2 drops
- **Indigestion** – Peppermint 2 drops, Sweet orange 4 drops and Coriander seed 4 drops
- **Emotional tension** – Neroli 2 drops, Palmarosa 4 drops and Mandarin 4 drops (This blend, halved, is particularly effective during pregnancy.)

## USING A HEAT PAD

After you have massaged in your blend, it is beneficial to apply heat to the area – this helps the skin to absorb the essential oils and also eases cramps or pain. Probably the easiest heat pad to use is a hot water bottle wrapped in a towel, but wheat bags, which can be heated in a micro-wave, are also good. Simply sit for a while with your heat pad over your abdomen and feel tension melt away.

# SELF-MASSAGE OF THE ABDOMEN ROUTINE

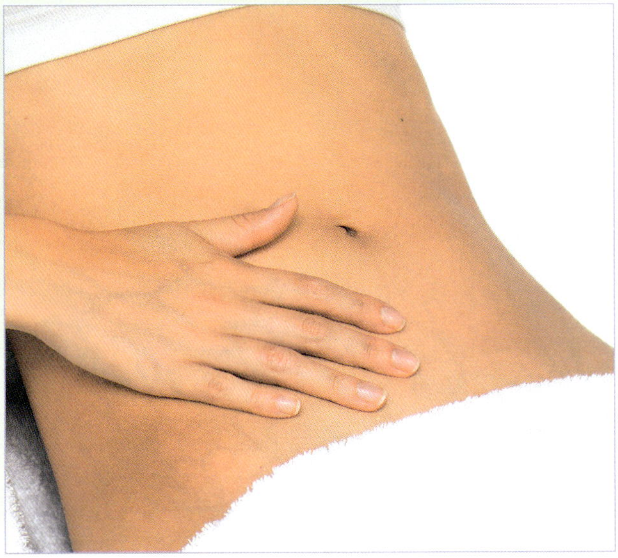

**1. Circle effleurage:** Using one hand, and starting at your right hip, slowly stroke up to under your breast, then over to the left side, down to your left hip and back to the beginning. Repeat several times.

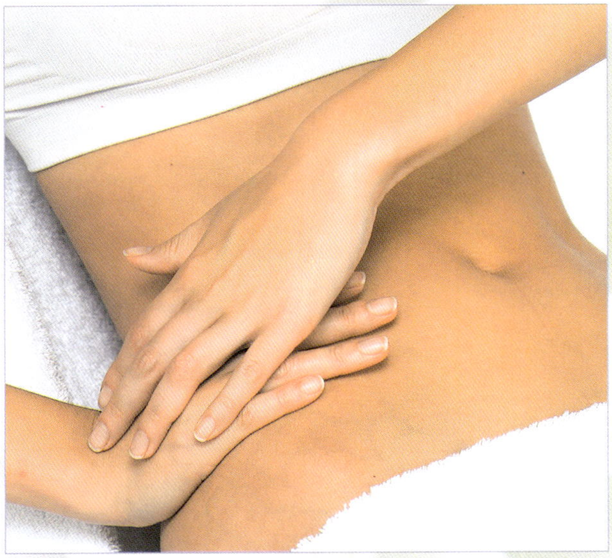

**2. Side-to-side stroking:** With one hand on top of the other, and starting at your right hip, slowly and gently stroke to the left side, across your abdomen, and back again, moving up toward your breast.

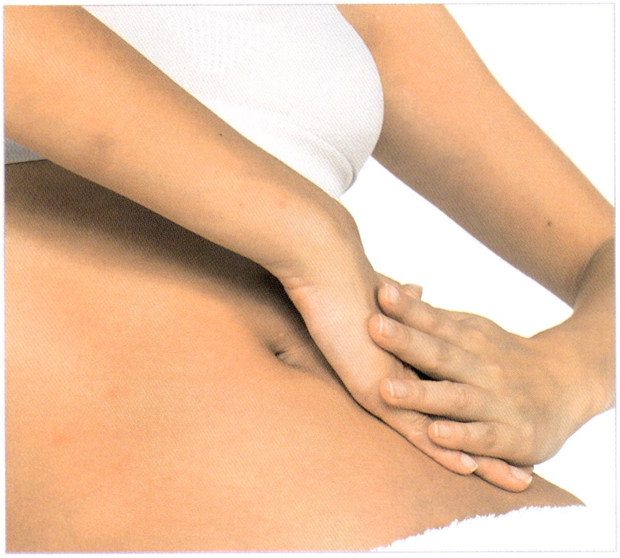

**3. Circle effleurage:** Repeat step 1 but this time make the movements really slowly and try to use slightly firmer pressure. By now your abdomen should be feeling very warm and relaxed.

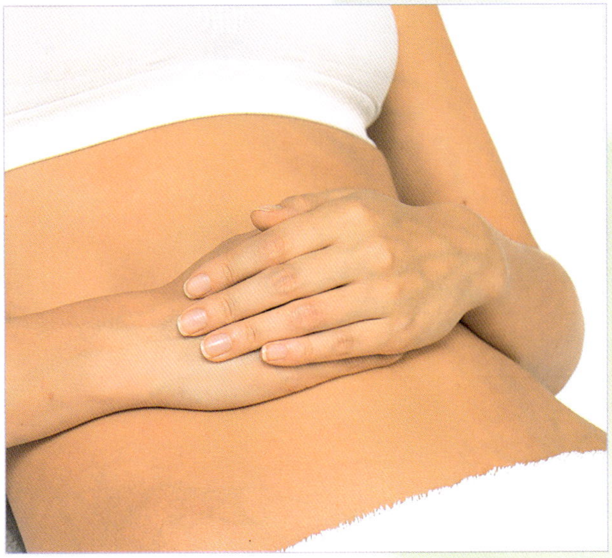

**4. Gentle rocking:** Bring both hands to a stop over your navel; gently rock the area from side to side three or four times. This tiny movement is very reassuring. Hold your hands still over your navel and feel the heat gather there.

# putting massage routines together

So far, we have been on a kind of journey through different parts of the body so that you can learn to massage different areas with appropriate techniques. You have also been using appropriate blends of essential oils to help particular areas. As you are learning it is good to concentrate on one area at a time, but the real art of massage lies in putting those massage routines together to make sequences.

Most of the routines you have learned so far will take up to 20 minutes at a time. However, if you want to give somebody a massage for an hour, you need to combine several sections to make a longer treatment. Here are some suggestions for putting massage routines together to create different, more complex sequences, which each last approximately one hour:

- **Face, décolletage, neck and shoulders** – this is a special treat for the face and nourishes the delicate skin of the chest area.
- **Back, neck and shoulders** – This sequence is a classic combination that is especially effective at releasing work-related stress and tension.
- **Face, neck and shoulders, abdomen** – This is a very relaxing sequence, which makes it an excellent massage to have in the evening.
- **Feet, legs, hands, arms, abdomen, neck and shoulders, back** – This body routine puts the emphasis on improving the circulation, particularly encouraging the blood flow back toward the heart. It makes a good daytime treatment. (Note that this sequence may take longer than one hour.)
- **Back, neck and shoulders, abdomen, arms, hands, legs and feet** – This body routine is good for relieving emotional stress and tiredness. It works by directing the awareness away from the head and down to the feet, and it is very relaxing to receive. (Note that this sequence may take longer than one hour.)

### CHOOSING AN APPROPRIATE AROMATHERAPY BLEND

If you decide to perform a more complex sequence, discuss with the person receiving which area(s) of their body they would most like you to treat – these should be the areas where they feel the most tension. Use this to guide you in your choice of oil blend. For example, if they feel that they are suffering mostly from tension in their back, go to the Back Massage section (pp.52–53), and choose a blend from that section. Usually 4tsp (20ml) of blend will be enough to massage both the back and the rest of the body too, but if the recipient is very large or has a lot of body hair you may need to make up double the quantity. The blend you choose will work for the whole body.

Aromatherapy massage is a highly creative therapy to practise. As you become increasingly confident and skilled in massage techniques, you will find that you are able to tailor your sequences and oils more effectively to help the different people that you massage.

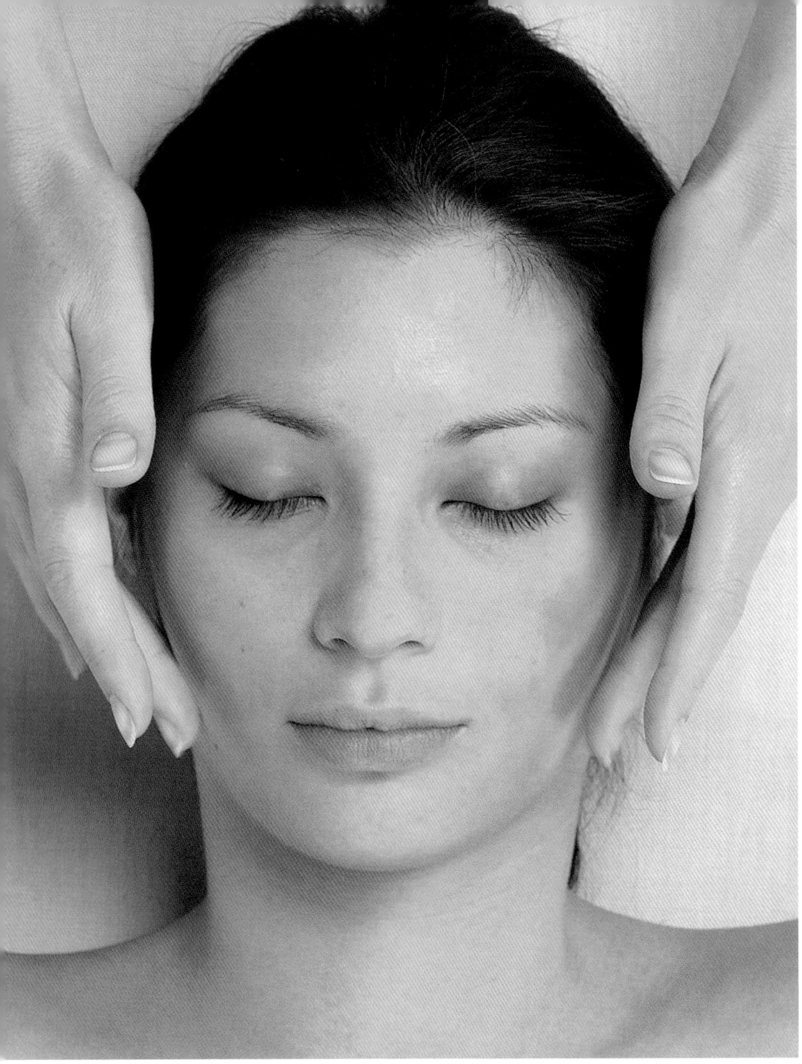
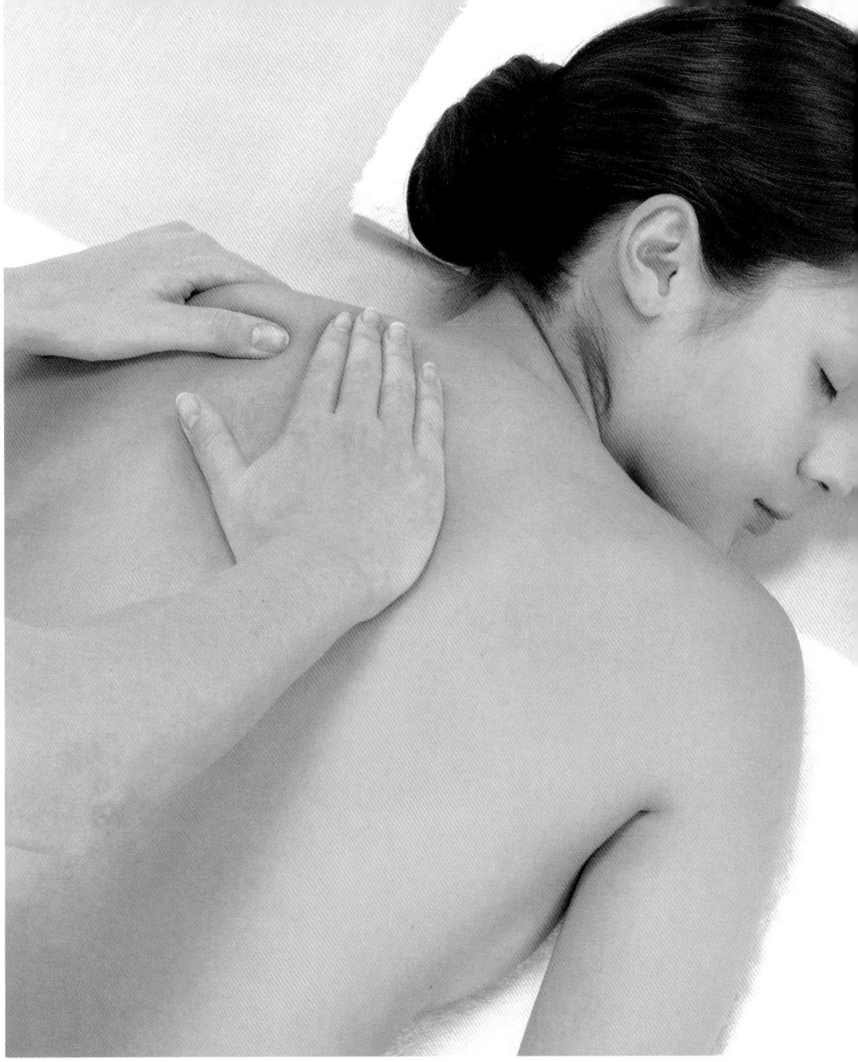
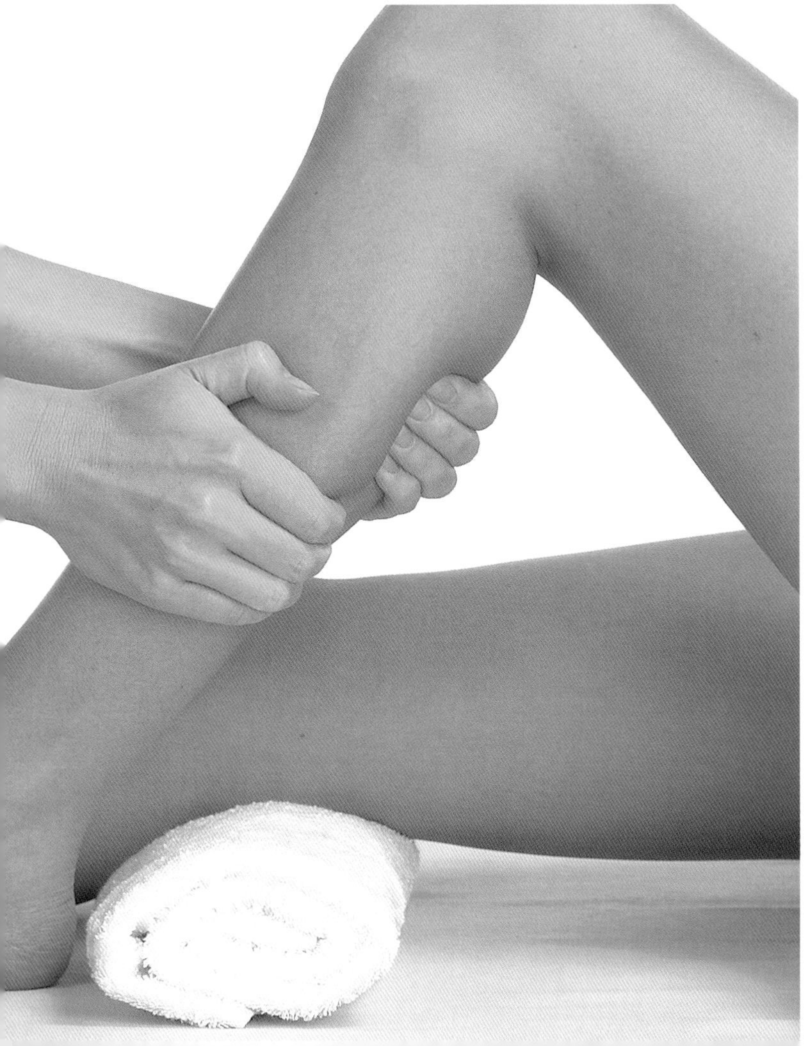
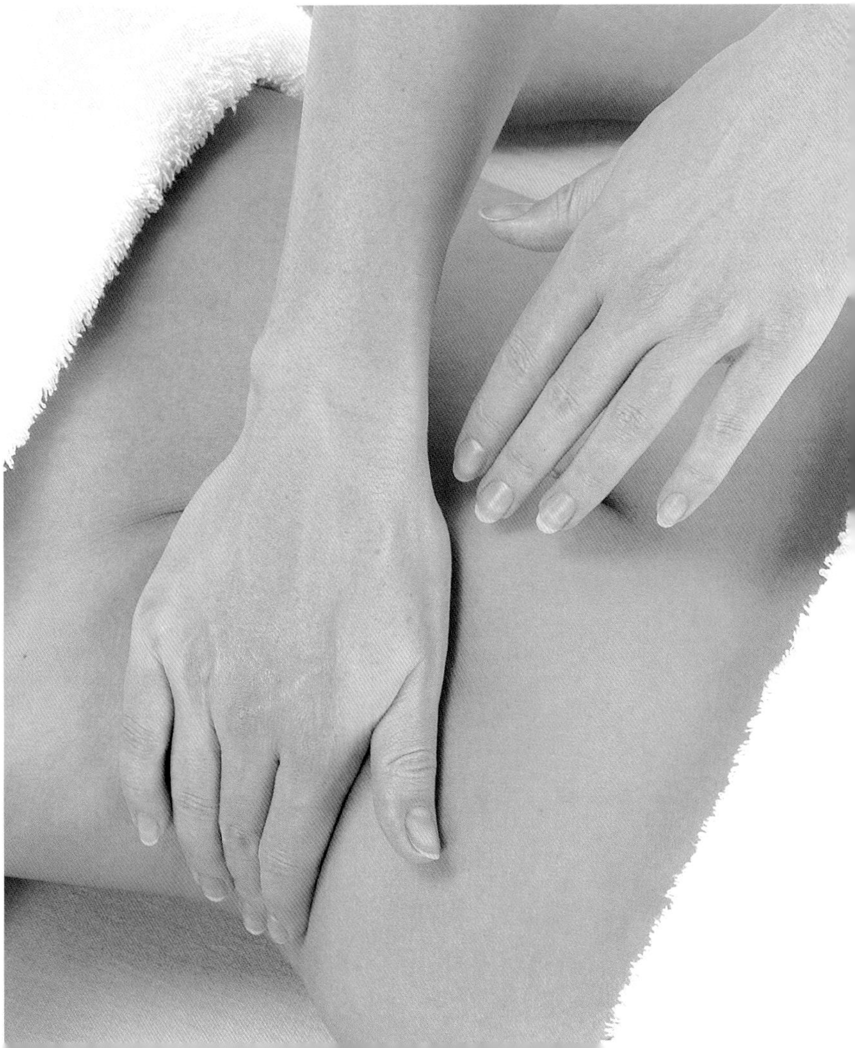

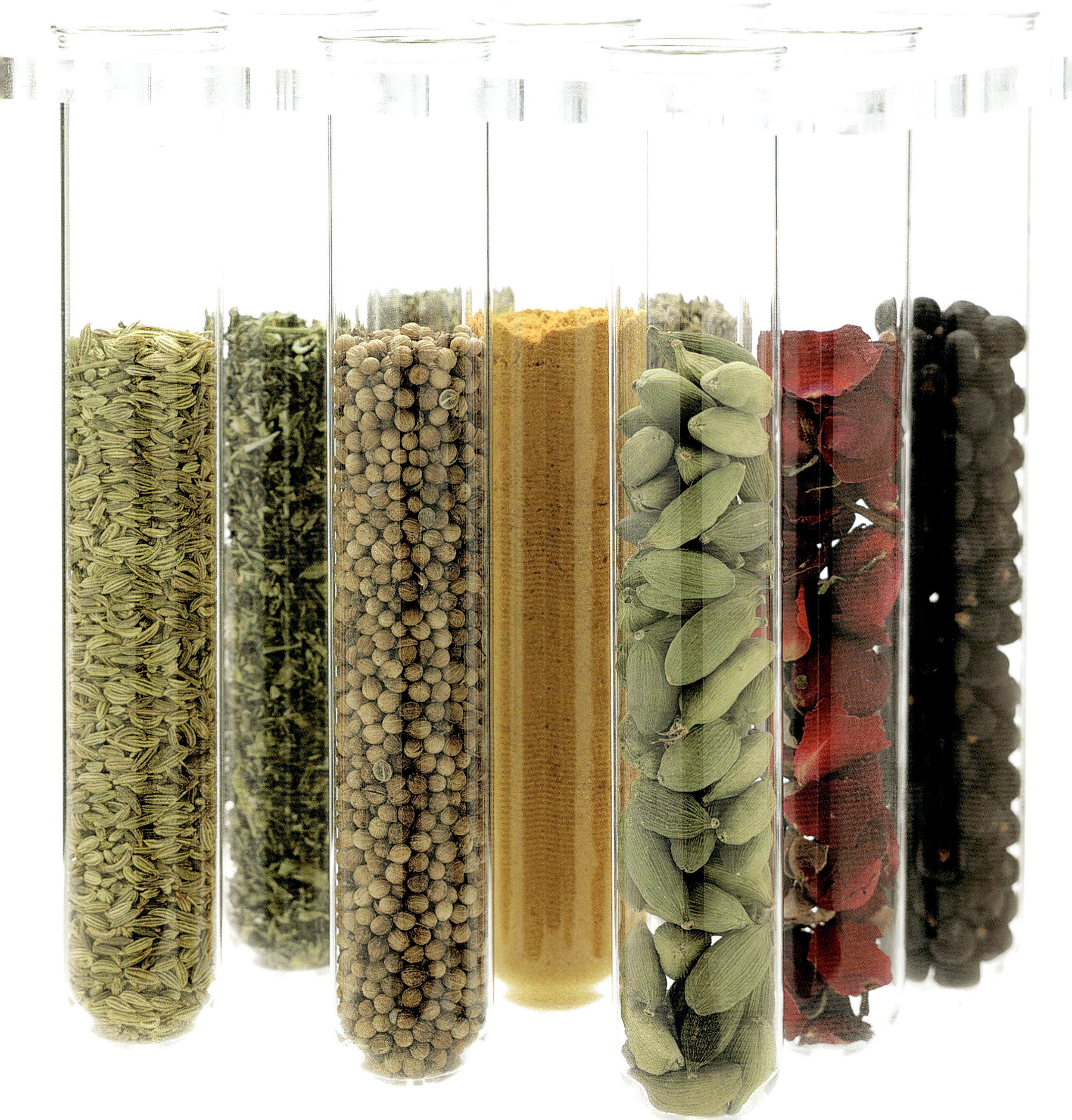

CHAPTER THREE

# essential oil directory

*This chapter presents 48 detailed profiles of individual essential oils, full of facts and tips for using them. The oils are divided into groups relating to the part of the plant from which each one is extracted, and comprise: flower oils; fruit, berry and seed oils; wood, resin and gum oils; and leaf and root oils.*

At the top of each page, next to the common name of the oil, the Latin name is given to identify the plant species that produces the essential oil. Next you will find a description of the fragrance of each oil, using perfumery terms, to guide you when buying an oil for the first time. Each profile continues by giving details of the oil's botanical source, what it looks like and where it is commonly found. You will also learn about the history and traditional uses of the plant, which are often linked to local culture. Next you will find out how each oil is extracted from the plant and how you should store it at home. I also explain the physical and psychological effects of the oil, and suggest a selection of blends for each one for you to use in your massage treatments. I conclude each profile with a note giving any relevant safety information.

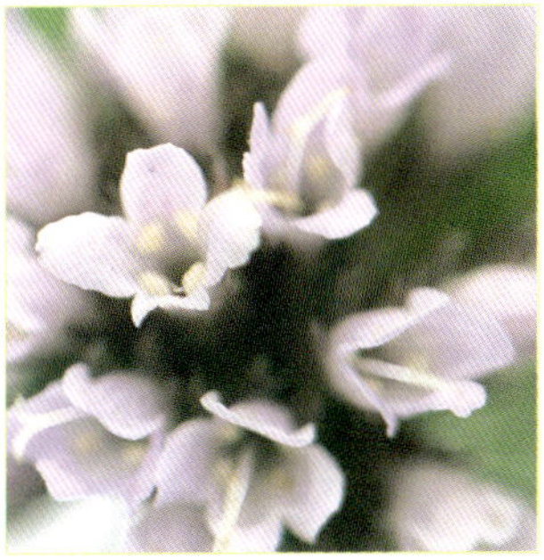

# flower oils

You only have to watch a bumble bee dive headlong into an aromatic, richly coloured rose at the height of summer to witness the power of essential oils in flowers. Precious and expensive, floral oils have a special place in aromatherapy, and the ones in this section represent a choice selection of the most sumptuous available.

When a bee nestles in a bloom what you are witnessing is the magnetic effect of the flower's aroma as it attracts the insect and invites it to seek out the nectar on offer in exchange for a dusting of pollen, which helps the flower to reproduce. Natural floral aromas are used as communication tools; over millennia some flowers have evolved fragrances that mimic the sex pheromones or scent of the particular moth or bee that visits it most. The aroma is released only when the plant flowers – a visual and aromatic advertisement to say that it is ready for reproduction.

The aromas found in flowers contain so many constituent parts that scientists find it difficult to identify them all – there can be hundreds of aromatic chemicals present at any one time. A perfumer I met some years ago told me that re-creating true floral aromas in their exact natural state using synthetic ingredients is almost impossible to achieve. I rather like that idea – nature still holds the upper hand, even against all our modern techniques of analysis.

Extracting the aromas – the essential oils – found in flowers is a painstaking and costly business, mainly because the oils are present only in tiny amounts. Steam distillation (see p.19) works for some flowers such as lavender, but may not be used for others because it evaporates too many of the delicate fragrance notes. Solvent extraction using petrochemicals is the only way to obtain aromatic compounds from fragile flowers such as jasmine.

The visual and aromatic effects of flowers can be extremely strong. Their colours make them attractive and lure you in to experience their aroma. Think of walking past a gorgeous rose bush covered in aromatic blooms one summer evening – you may stop in your tracks almost without realizing it. Over the many years that I have practised aromatherapy, I have found myself becoming increasingly sensitive to natural aromas in the outdoors, to the point where I simply have to follow an aromatic signal just to find out what it is!

Aromatherapists treat floral oils with great respect, aware that just the tiniest amount can help to create a fabulous blend. When these are massaged into the body the recipient will feel incredibly nurtured. Floral aromas have soothing and calming effects on the mind as well as the body, and blends created with floral essential oils can also trigger positive mental associations because flowers bloom in summer, which is often a time when we feel most relaxed and happy.

The gentle sweetness of flowers also helps to soothe fraught emotions, bringing a sense of peace and tranquillity to both the person giving and the person receiving the massage treatment.

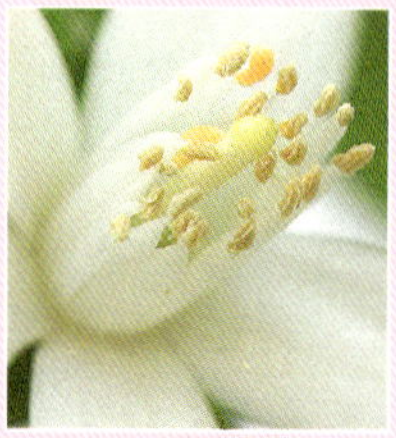

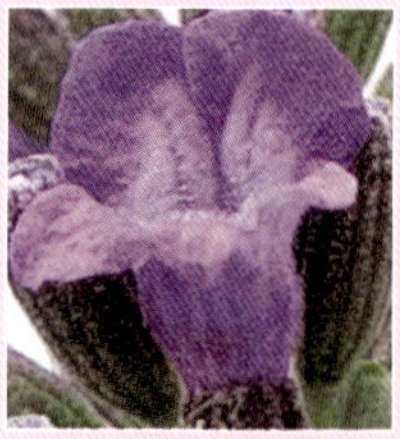

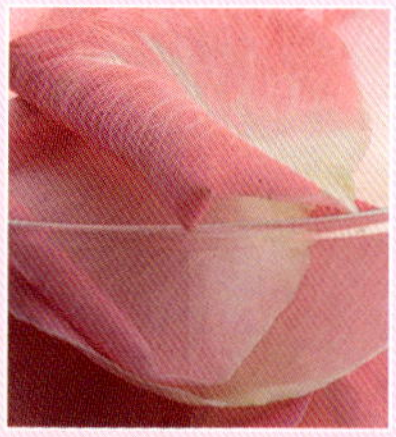

# roman chamomile *Anthemis nobilis*

Roman chamomile has a sweet, fruity and herbaceous aroma, very light and pleasant, with underlying notes rather like fresh hay. In tiny amounts there is an apple-like fragrance, which is subtle and fresh.

### Botanical source and background

A member of the extensive Compositae (Asteraceae) family, Roman chamomile is native to western Europe and grows wild in many countries. It is cultivated commercially for its oil in the UK, France and Hungary. It has feathery green foliage with round white flowers on single erect stems, and grows up to 12in (30cm) tall. Roman chamomile is one of the oldest known medicinal herbs; in Ancient Egypt it was used as a cure for fever. The name "chamomile" comes from the Greek words *kamai*, meaning "on the ground", and *melon*, meaning "apple" – in other words, a low-growing plant, smelling of apples! It was used by the 17th-century English herbalist Nicholas Culpeper, to tone the liver, stomach and spleen, and to help relieve headaches.

### Extraction and storage

Steam distillation of Roman chamomile flowers and stalks yields a very pale blue or greenish-blue essential oil. The colour comes from a blue constituent in the plant called azulene, which has anti-inflammatory properties. In the refrigerator the essential oil will keep for up to two years; at cool room temperature (54°F/12°C) up to one year.

### Physical and psychological effects

*Anti-inflammatory:* soothes irritated, sore skin and inflamed sunburn
*Skin-healing:* heals damaged skin, eczema or psoriasis
*Antispasmodic:* soothes stomach cramps, aches or colicky pains
*Digestive tonic:* stimulates the digestion of fatty foods and eases indigestion or nausea
*Nervous restorative:* soothes fraught nerves, irritability or anxiety; helps relieve insomnia

### Special Roman chamomile blends, in 4tsp (20ml) carrier oil

*Skin-healer:* Roman chamomile 4 drops, Lavender 4 drops, Palmarosa 2 drops
*Digestive tonic:* Roman chamomile 4 drops, Mandarin 4 drops, Ginger 2 drops
*Mental-soother:* Roman chamomile 4 drops, Sandalwood 4 drops, Neroli 2 drops

### Safety information

Very rarely, people have experienced skin sensitivity to Roman chamomile essential oil but it is generally non-toxic and non-irritating.

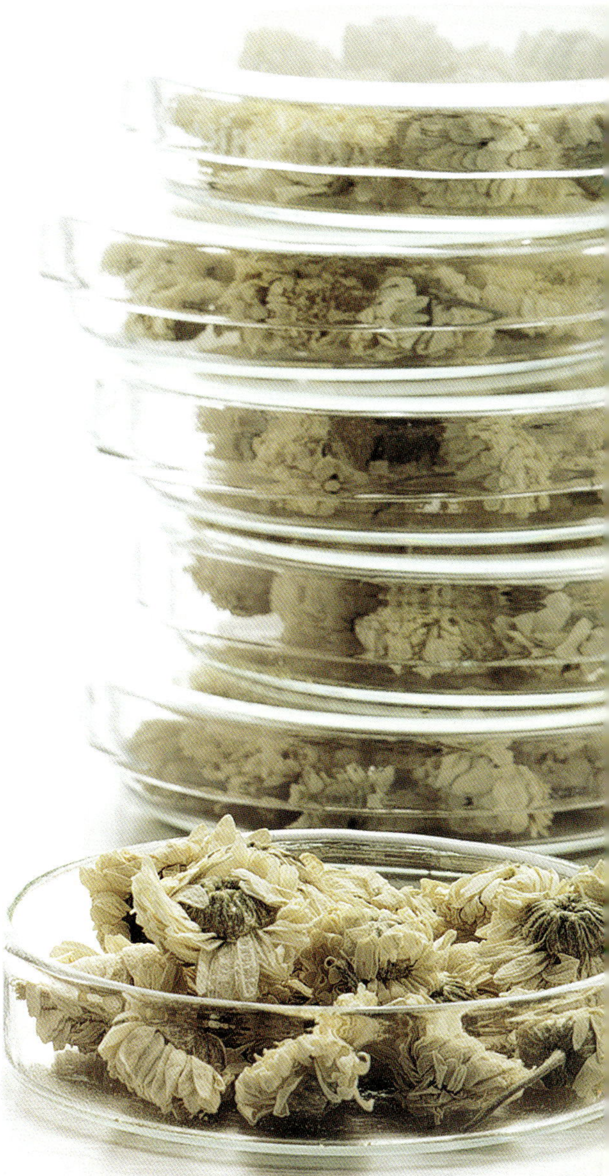

# ylang ylang *Cananga odorata*

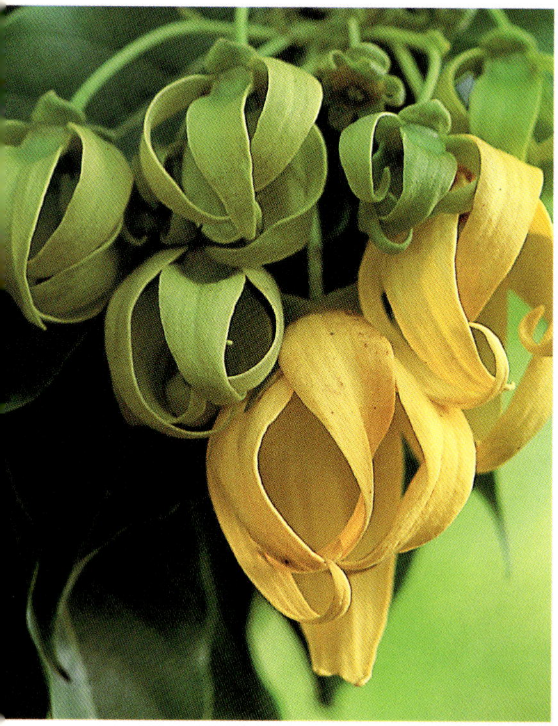

Ylang ylang has an intensely sweet floral fragrance and is heady and exotic, with a hint of musk and spice as it evaporates. It lasts for a long time on the skin, leaving a sensual and subtle aroma of tropical flowers.

### Botanical source and background

Ylang ylang belongs to the Annonaceae plant family and is originally native to Southeast Asia. The oil is produced in Indonesia, the Philippines, Java, Madagascar and Réunion. It is an evergreen tropical tree up to 60ft (20m) tall, with large fragrant yellow, pink or mauve flowers; the yellow blooms are picked for distillation as they are considered to have the finest fragrance. In Indonesia, the flowers are strewn on the beds of newly married couples. Ylang ylang flowers steeped in coconut oil are a traditional tropical remedy for fevers, malaria, insect bites and infections, and are used to condition the skin or hair. The Victorians used ylang ylang in the formula "Macassar oil", a popular hair tonic.

### Extraction and storage

Ylang ylang distillation uses freshly picked flowers and is a slow process. Essential oil is drawn off four times, giving four grades of oil known as Extra, 1, 2 and 3. Ylang ylang Extra, used for aromatherapy, is the best quality; the other grades are used in the perfumery industry. In the refrigerator ylang ylang will last up to two years; at cool room temperature (54°F/12°C), up to one year.

### Physical and emotional effects

*Skin-toning:* a tonic for all skin types, particularly oily or combination, and the hair and scalp
*Hypotensive:* helps lower high blood pressure
*Antidepressant:* eases irritability and frustrated feelings, such as those common with PMS
*Aphrodisiac:* melts frozen emotions between partners
*Nervous relaxant:* relaxes the mind and nervous system; helps epileptics manage seizures.

### Special ylang ylang blends, in 4tsp (20ml) carrier oil

*Oily/combination skin tonic:* Ylang ylang 1 drop, Patchouli 1 drop, Frankincense 3 drops
*Antidepressant:* Ylang ylang 2 drops, Sweet orange 4 drops, Sandalwood 4 drops
*Mental-rejuvenator:* Ylang ylang 2 drops, May chang 4 drops, Mandarin 4 drops

### Safety information

People occasionally report headaches because of the strong floral aroma; avoid with headache or migraine sufferers. Also, avoid on sensitive or damaged skin.

# neroli *Citrus x aurantium var. amara*

Neroli, also called orange blossom, has a balanced aroma of bitter-sweet citrus notes mixed with sweet floral tones, becoming rich and soft as it evaporates. It lasts a long time on the skin, with a gentle, sweet fragrance.

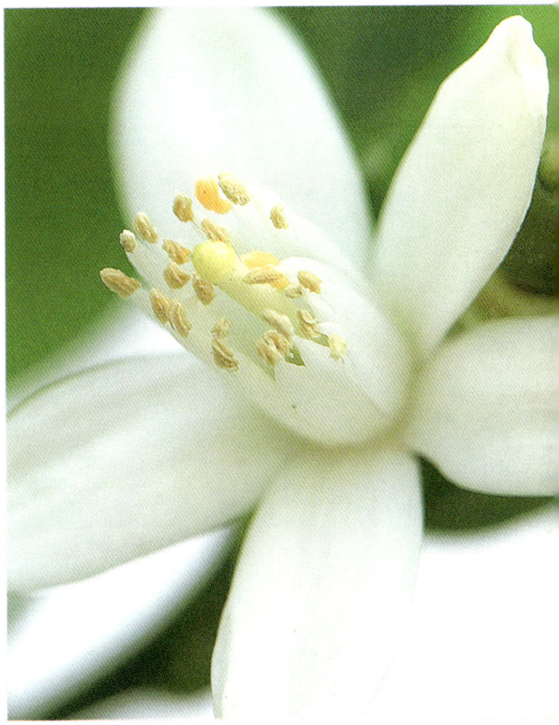

### Botanical source and background

Neroli essential oil, produced in southern France, Morocco, Tunisia and Italy, comes from the flowers of the bitter orange tree, which is a member of the Rutaceae family. It is an evergreen, growing up to 30ft (10m), with glossy green leaves. Its flowers are creamy white and swell into oranges with a wrinkled skin. The bitter orange flowers in May, and blossoms are picked two or three times a week, at sunrise, to preserve their aroma. The name "neroli" is linked to an Italian princess of Nerola who used the oil to perfume her gloves. Along with bergamot, lavender and rosemary essential oils, neroli oil an ingredient of eau-de-Cologne. In southern Europe, neroli flowers are often added to bridal bouquets.

### Extraction and storage

Steam distillation of the flowers yields both a pale yellow essential oil and orange flower water, which is excellent for skin-freshening. Around 220lbs (100kgs) of neroli flowers will yield approximately 3⅓lbs (1.5kgs) of essential oil. This will last for two years if kept in the refrigerator, and one year kept at cool room temperature (54°F/12°C).

### Physical and psychological effects

*Antispasmodic:* calms indigestion, stomach cramps, nausea and irritable bowel symptoms, especially those made worse by stress, in both adults and children
*Skin-healing:* improves mature or very dry skin and rejuvenates the complexion; highly recommended for facial treatments
*Nervous restorative:* soothes nervous tension, fear and emotional stress
*Sedative:* eases shock and hysteria, and calms anxiety attacks

### Special neroli blends, in 4tsp (20ml) carrier oil

*Mood-enhancer:* Neroli 2 drops, Palmarosa 4 drops, Lemon 4 drops
*Mature facial tonic:* Neroli 1 drop, Patchouli 2 drops, Sandalwood 2 drops
*Stomach-soother:* Neroli 2 drops, Cardamom 2 drops, Sweet orange 6 drops

### Safety information

Neroli oil is non-sensitizing, non-toxic and non-irritating.

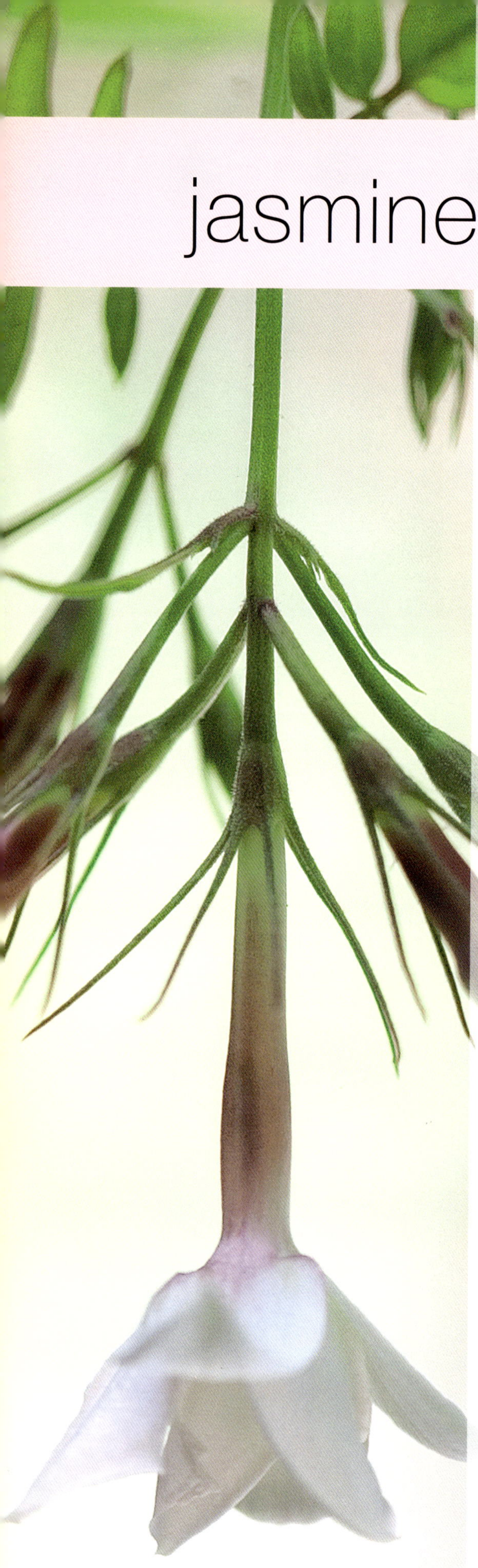

# jasmine absolute *Jasminum officinale*

Jasmine absolute has an intense rich sweet floral aroma, and is musky and soft as it evaporates. It is heady almost to the point of being intoxicating, and lingers on the skin with a subtle and exotic perfume.

### Botanical source and background

*Jasminum officiale* belongs to the plant family Oleaceae and is an attractive climber growing up to 30ft (10m) tall. It has delicate, pointed, dark green leaves and tiny white star-shaped flowers, which are particularly aromatic at dusk. Another jasmine species, *Jasminum sambac*, from southern India, yields an absolute with an even richer aroma. In India, wreaths of jasmine flowers are worn at weddings, and the flower is known as "queen of the night" because its fragrance is stronger after dusk. Jasmine absolute used to be produced primarily in the south of France but, today, most of it comes from Morocco.

### Extraction and storage

Because jasmine flowers are too fragile for distillation, chemical solvents are used to dissolve the aroma from the petals, eventually producing a reddish-orange absolute. Around 2200lbs (1,000kgs) of flowers is needed to produce 3⅓lbs (1.5kgs) of oil. It will keep for two years in the refrigerator or one year at cool room temperature (54°F/12°C).

### Physical and psychological effects

*Skin-healing:* restores dry, wrinkled or sagging skin; improves skin elasticity
*Menstrual tonic:* regulates painful or heavy periods – use in abdominal massage late in the cycle
*Aphrodisiac:* improves low sexual vitality and encourages harmony in relationships
*Nervous restorative:* improves low self-esteem and mental anxiety

### Special jasmine blends, in 4tsp (20ml) carrier oil

*Deluxe facial care:* Jasmine 1 drop, Frankincense 1 drop, Neroli 2 drops, Rose 1 drop
*Menstrual-soother:* Jasmine 2 drops, Rosewood 4 drops, Myrrh 4 drops
*Emotional support:* Jasmine 2 drops, Sweet orange 4 drops, Sandalwood 4 drops

### Safety information

Do not use on allergy-prone skin. Because of its intense floral aroma, jasmine oil is not recommended for people who regularly suffer from migraines or headaches.

# lavender *Lavandula angustifolia*

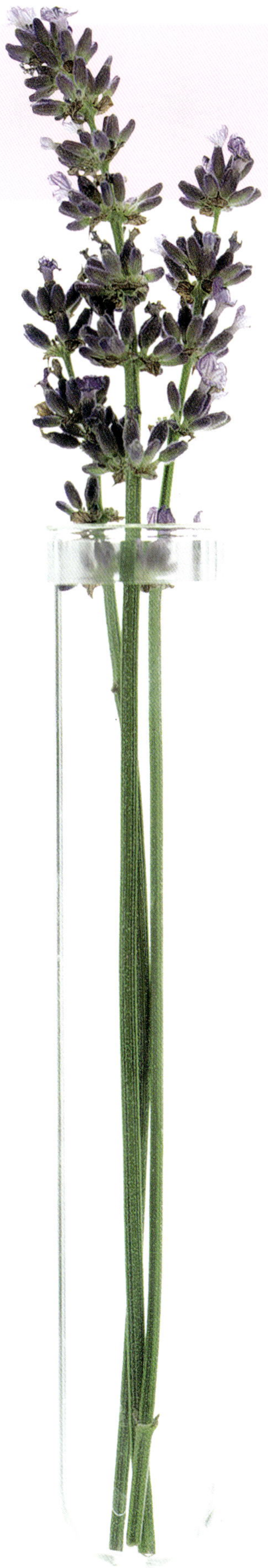

Lavender essential oil is generally sweet and fresh with soft, warm and pungent underlying notes. Depending on its country of origin, the aroma will range from floral and sweet to sharp and medicinal.

### Botanical source and background

Lavender is a member of the plant family Labiatae (Lamiaceae), which includes many common herbs. It is a bushy evergreen shrub, up to 3ft (1m) in height, with green or grey-green leaves. In summer, it produces tall stalks and compact heads of purple or purple-blue flowers. The name lavender is linked to the Latin *lavare*, which means to wash, because its fresh smell is associated with cleanliness. The Romans took lavender as far north as England where, by the 16th century, it became a common plant in cottage gardens. In the early 20th century, French perfume chemist René Gattefosse discovered the healing properties of lavender oil when treating a laboratory burn on his hand (see p.15).

### Extraction and storage

Steam distillation of the flowers and stalks yields a pale, colourless essential oil, as well as lavender water, which is a traditional skin-freshener. Lavender harvested from 1 acre (0.5ha) of land produces about 12lbs (5.5kgs) of essential oil. If kept in the refrigerator, it will last up to two years; stored at cool room temperature (54°F/12°C), up to one year.

### Physical and psychological effects

*Wound-healing:* helps to heal cuts, grazes and wounds, especially when combined with tea tree oil (see p.128)
*Skin-healing:* repairs skin damaged by sunburn, burns or eczema
*Analgesic:* eases the pain of burns or scalds – apply two drops neat on a cotton wool pad
*Antispasmodic:* helps muscular aches, pains and stiffness, and eases menstrual cramps
*Respiratory tonic:* soothes the respiratory passages, helps colds or chesty coughs
*Nervous restorative:* calms nervous tension, exhaustion and mental stress

### Special lavender blends, in 4tsp (20ml) carrier oil

*Skin-healer:* Lavender 4 drops, Myrrh 2 drops, Tea tree 4 drops
*Respiratory tonic:* Lavender 4 drops, Cardamom 4 drops, Lemon 2 drops
*Stress-reliever:* Lavender 4 drops, Neroli 2 drops, Rosewood 4 drops

### Safety information

Lavender oil is non-irritant, non-toxic and non-sensitizing.

# lavendin *Lavandula x intermedia*

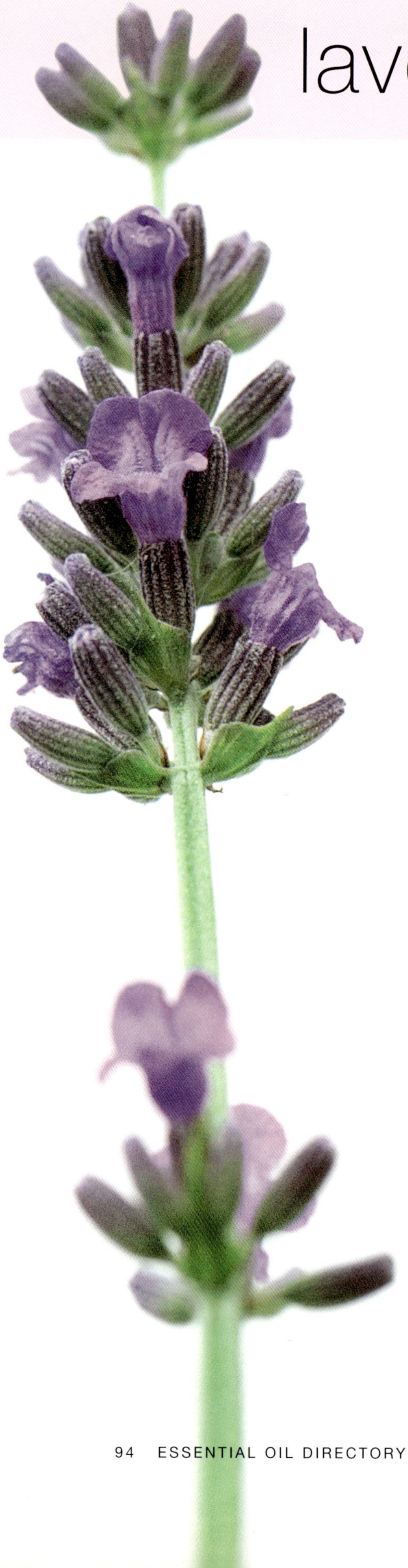

Lavendin essential oil has greater pungency than true lavender, and is sharp and fresh, with sweeter, woody undertones. Its medicinal fragrance often makes it more acceptable to men than the more floral true lavender.

### Botanical source and background

Like true lavender, lavendin is a member of the plant family Labiatae (Lamiaceae). It is mainly grown in southern France, Hungary, Spain and Croatia. A hybrid cross between *Lavandula angustifolia* (true lavender) and *Lavandula latifolia* (spike lavender), lavendin grows up to 4ft (1.2m) tall, and has stiff four-sided stems and flower heads up to 2in (5cm) in length. Lavendin flowers are usually purple, but a fragrant white variety is also available. Its aroma is stronger and more pungent than true lavender. Lavendin produces a higher yield of essential oil than true lavender and is used to make perfumes, soaps and toiletries. Spike lavender was well known to the Romans as a respiratory tonic; in the 1st century CE Dioscorides listed it in his *Herbal*, a standard medical textbook for more than 500 years.

### Extraction and storage

Steam distillation of the flowers and stalks yields a pale, almost colourless essential oil. If kept in the refrigerator, lavendin essential oil will last up to two years, if stored at cool room temperature (54°F/12°C), it will keep for up to a year.

### Physical and psychological effects

*Antispasmodic:* helps stiff aching tight muscles, backache or strains after sports
*Analgesic:* pain-relieving for muscular strains, cramps and arthritic stiffness
*Circulatory tonic:* improves poor circulation, warms cold hands and feet
*General tonic:* recommended as a spring tonic after the winter to encourage detoxification
*Respiratory tonic:* eases coughs, colds and respiratory problems
*Mentally-rejuvenating:* refreshes the brain and improves poor concentration

### Special lavendin blends, in 4tsp (20ml) carrier oil

*Muscular aches:* Lavendin 4 drops, Myrtle 4 drops, Black pepper 2 drops
*Spring tonic:* Lavendin 4 drops, Fennel 4 drops, Lemon 2 drops
*Mental uplift:* Lavendin 4 drops, Grapefruit 4 drops, Peppermint 2 drops

### Safety information

Do not use lavendin on epilepsy sufferers; it has a very different chemical composition to true lavender, and is much stronger and more mentally stimulating.

# german chamomile *Matricaria chamomilla*

German chamomile essential oil has a warm, deep camphoraceous aroma: bitter and herbaceous, with sweeter, earthy notes as it evaporates. An extremely pungent fragrance, your blends need only a small amount.

### Botanical source and background

German chamomile belongs to the large Compositae (Asteraceae) plant family. It is commercially produced in Germany, Hungary and other Eastern European countries. It has broad flowers with defined white petals and golden yellow centres growing on tall stems, up to 18in (50cm) high, with feathery, dark green leaves. German chamomile is a traditional herbal remedy for headaches and migraines. The Anglo-Saxons called it "maythen" and revered it as one of their nine most healing herbs. In medieval times, dried chamomile flowers were used to scent linen and fragrance rooms. German chamomile is the species of chamomile used as a herbal tea (particularly in Europe) to help stomach aches, fevers, indigestion and nervous tension.

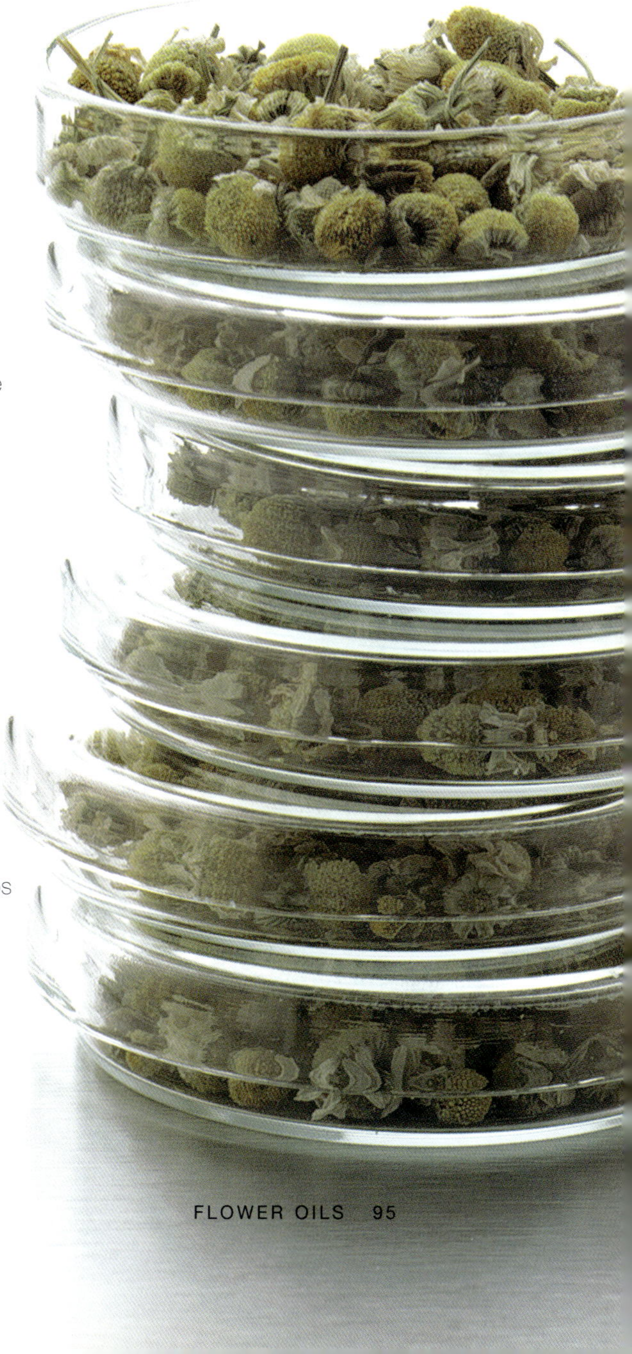

### Extraction and storage

Steam distillation of the flowers yields a tiny quantity of deep blue essential oil, coloured by the constituent azulene. Because of the small yield, German chamomile is much more expensive than Roman chamomile. It will keep for up to two years in the refrigerator, or up to one year at cool room temperature (54°F/12°C).

### Physical and emotional effects

*Anti-inflammatory:* calms reddened, itching or inflamed skin
*Skin-healing:* heals wounded or deeply cracked skin
*Sedative:* helps relieve insomnia, restlessness and stress
*Antispasmodic:* eases cramping pains such as indigestion or menstrual spasms
*Analgesic:* eases backache, muscular tension, stiffness and arthritic pain

### Special German chamomile blends, in 4tsp (20ml) carrier oil

*Skin-healer:* German chamomile 2 drops, Myrrh 4 drops, Frankincense 4 drops
*Menstrual-soother:* German chamomile 2 drops, Sweet marjoram 4 drops, Ginger 4 drops
*Children's insomnia blend (for ages 3 to 10):* German chamomile 1 drop, Lavender 2 drops, Neroli 1 drop.

### Safety information

German chamomile essential oil is non-toxic, non-irritating and non-sensitizing.

# rose *Rosa damascena, Rosa centifolia*

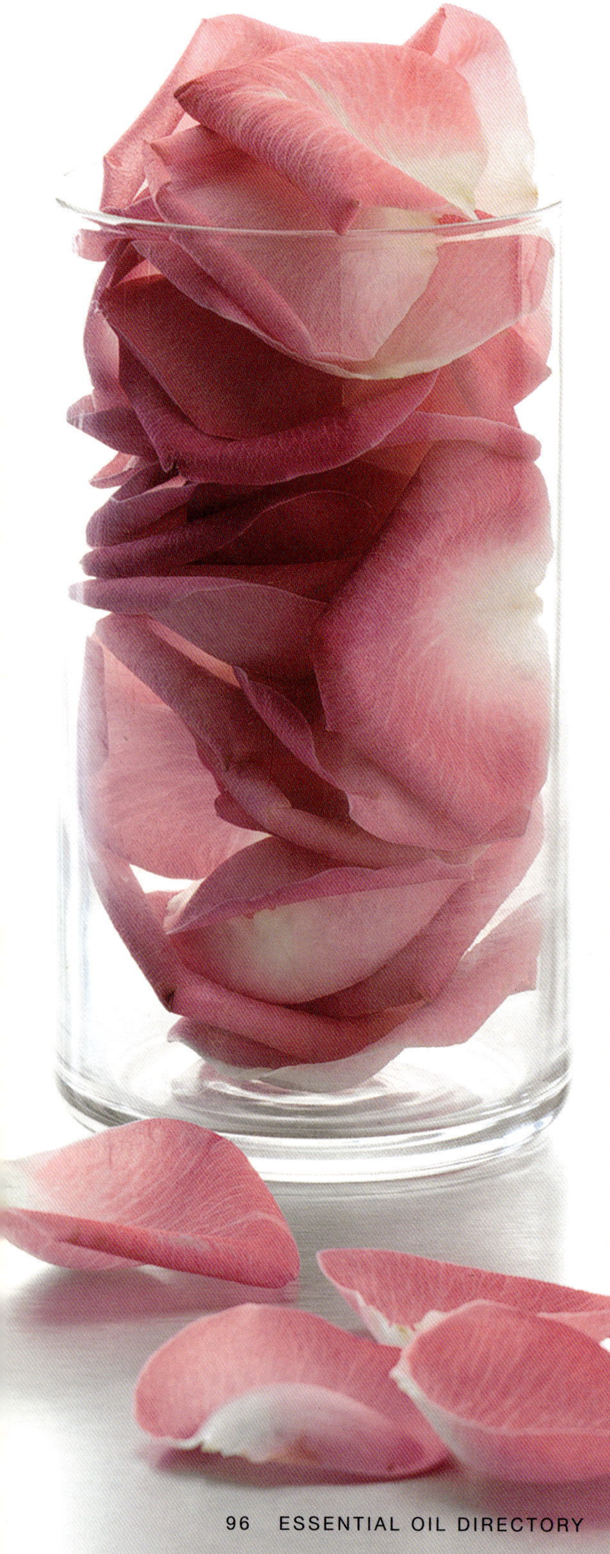

There are two types of rose essential oil: otto, from the *Rosa damascena* flower, has a soft, sweet aroma, reminiscent of honey with a hint of citrus; absolute, from *Rosa centifolia*, is stronger and musky with rich, sweet notes.

### Botanical source and background

Both are members of the plant family Rosaceae. *Rosa damascena* (the damask rose) is grown mostly in Bulgaria, and *Rosa centifolia* (the cabbage rose) in Turkey and Morocco. The damask flower is small, with just three or four rows of petals, while the cabbage bloom is larger and round, with dense layerings of fine petals. Both bushes grow to around 6ft (2m). Originally from China, these roses were revered by the ancient Greeks, Romans and Arabs, and have been used for thousands of years in cosmetics, perfumery and medicine.

### Extraction and storage

Steam distillation produces the almost colourless rose otto ("rose oil") from the damask rose. Solvent extraction is used to produce the yellow-orange coloured rose absolute from *centifolia* flowers. If stored in the refrigerator, both otto and absolute will keep for up to two years; at a cool room temperature of around 54°F (12°C), they will last one year. If the otto solidifies in the refrigerator, warm the bottle in your hands to liquefy it.

### Physical and psychological effects

*Anti-inflammatory:* rose otto soothes inflamed or irritated skin, itching and soreness and repairs damage from burns
*Hydrating:* both rose otto and absolute hydrate and soften the skin, improving dry or mature complexions, and those damaged by sun or wind
*Skin-toning:* rose absolute has a slightly astringent effect on facial skin, tightening pores and improving the appearance of visible veins
*Hormone-balancing:* using rose otto or absolute in massage twice during the menstrual cycle can help to ease pre-menstrual symptoms such as fluid retention

### Special rose blends, in 4tsp (20ml) carrier oil

*Dry/mature skin facial:* Rose otto 1 drop, Sandalwood 2 drops, Frankincense 2 drops
*Emotional-soother:* Rose absolute 2 drops, Lemon 4 drops, Myrtle 4 drops
*Hormone-balancer:* Rose otto 2 drops, Clary sage 4 drops, Sweet orange 4 drops

### Safety information

Both rose otto and absolute are non-toxic, non-irritant and non-sensitizing.

# clary sage *Salvia sclarea*

Clary sage essential oil has a rich, musky and nutty fragrance with sweet woody undertones. Powerful and pungent, it is often used in perfumery to "fix" a blend, giving it a long-lasting aroma.

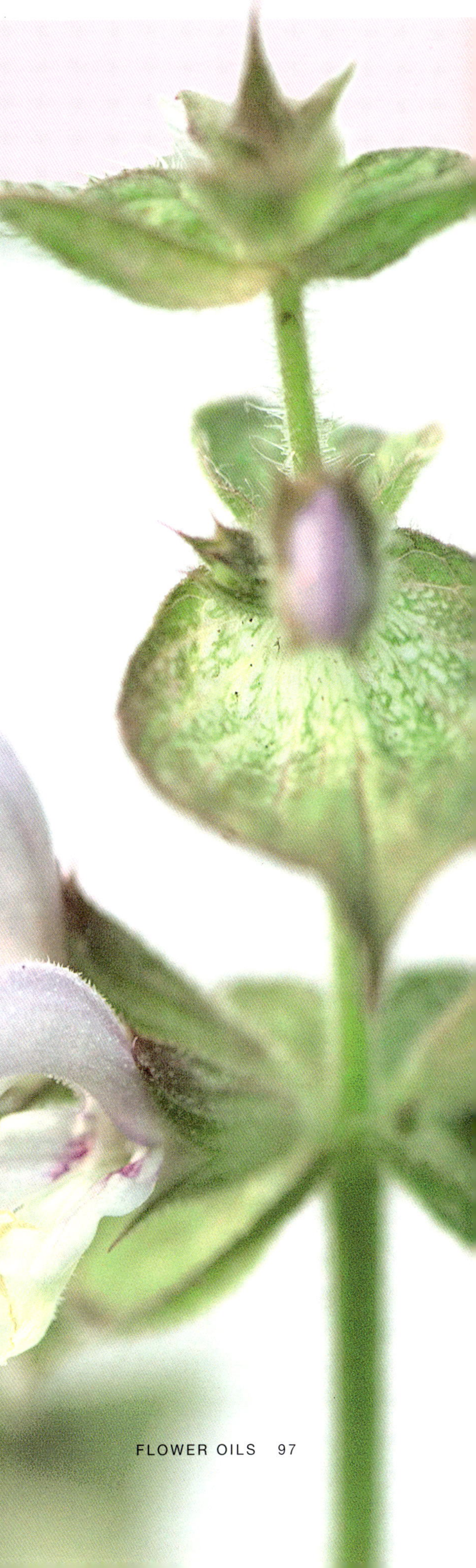

### Botanical source and background

A member of the plant family Labiatae (Lamiaceae), clary sage is originally native to southern Europe. It is now produced commercially in France, Morocco, the US and the UK. It is the giant of the sages with large pointed and hairy leaves at its base, and tall stalks up to 4ft (1.2m), with attractive pinkish-blue flowers. The whole plant is highly aromatic with a powerful musky fragrance. The flowering stalks are cut in the summer for essential oil production. An old French name for the plant is *toute bonne*, which means "good for everything". The English name "clary" is a corruption of "clear eye", a reference to the traditional use of the seeds as an eye tonic – they release a gel-like substance when soaked in water, which was used as an eye wash. In the 17th century, the herbalist Culpeper used the leaves boiled in vinegar and mixed with honey to help skin infections.

### Extraction and storage

Steam distillation of the flowers and stalks yields a pale yellow oil, which will last up to two years in the refrigerator, and up to one year at cool room temperature (54°F/12°C).

### Physical and psychological effects

*Skin-balancing:* regulates excessively oily or combination skins; also tones greasy scalps
*Antispasmodic:* eases asthmatic symptoms by calming and slowing the breath
*Hormone-balancing:* regulates the hormones, particularly helpful for pre-menstrual symptoms and menstrual cramps
*Antidepressant:* uplifts negative moods, easing anxiety and emotional stress
*Nervous restorative:* soothes fraught and overstretched nerves

### Special clary sage blends, in 4tsp (20ml) carrier oil

*Oily-skin treat:* Clary sage 1 drop, Cypress 2 drops, Lemon 2 drops
*Hormone-balancer:* Clary sage 2 drops, Rose otto 2 drops, Sandalwood 6 drops
*Nerve tonic:* Clary sage 2 drops, Rosewood 4 drops, Myrtle 4 drops
*Antidepressant:* Clary sage 2 drops, Mandarin 4 drops, Frankincense 4 drops

### Safety information

Clary sage essential oil is non-toxic, non-sensitizing and non-irritating.

# fruit, berry and seed oils

This group of essential oils are found in the end-products of the flowering process – fruits, berries and seeds. They all have powerful cleansing effects that have been used for culinary and medicinal purposes as well as in aromatherapy massage.

The fruits, berries and seeds in this section have evolved in many special ways to attract different types of animal or bird to ingest them, or transport them away to different sites where they will produce new plants. Their aromatic compounds make them taste and smell better to animals and birds than other nearby plant life, so they are more likely to be chosen and eaten. Essential oils extracted from these sources often have stimulating effects on digestive processes and liver function.

One of the most obvious groups of fruits from which essential oils are extracted is the Rutaceae family. These are brightly coloured fruit such as the mandarin, sweet orange, lemon and grapefruit. They are attractive to the eye, and their peel contains tiny globular sacs filled with citrus essential oils. As the fruit is eaten, a small amount of the oil is released, adding to the flavour and filling the air with zesty aromas. Mouth-wateringly fresh, these fruits are associated with summer and brightness – as essential oils they are some of the most popular in aromatherapy.

Berries are smaller versions of fruit; juniper berries, black peppercorns, nutmeg, and cardamom pods are spicy, pungent and fragrant examples, which become even more fragrant as they dry in the sun. These spices have been used for thousands of years in systems of medicine such as the Ayurvedic tradition in India, where food and medicine are completely interlinked and the spices play a vital role in maintaining digestion and supporting the immune system.

The Umbelliferae plant family is the source of some important seed essential oils such as coriander, carrot, fennel and cumin. These have been used in traditional Western herbalism for centuries – as digestive, kidney and liver tonics. The essential oils from these seeds are pungent and have a slight hint of aniseed in their fragrances. Historically, famous herbalists, such as Nicholas Culpeper in the 17th century, praised these plants for having many virtues, including being able to dissolve deposits such as kidney stones.

In aromatherapy massage we frequently work to stimulate the system to detoxify itself; many massage movements, for example those performed on the legs, are designed to encourage the lymphatic system to rid the body of excess fluid. By using a massage blend containing essential oils from the fruit, berry or seed groups the recipient benefits from both the massage strokes themselves and the powerful cleansing effects of the essential oils. You can see the results quite quickly – it is not uncommon for people receiving massage to need to visit the bathroom very soon after treatment! With their toning and purifying effects, oils from these groups are excellent for spa-style treatments or anti-cellulite massage. They also make great springtime blends to wake up the system after the winter.

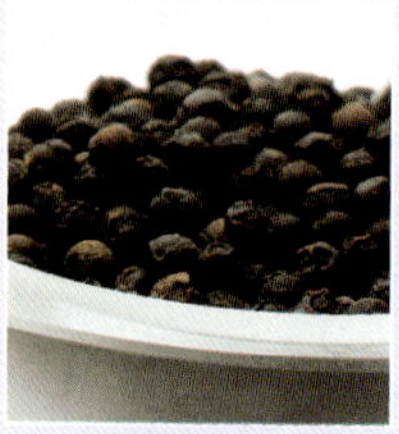
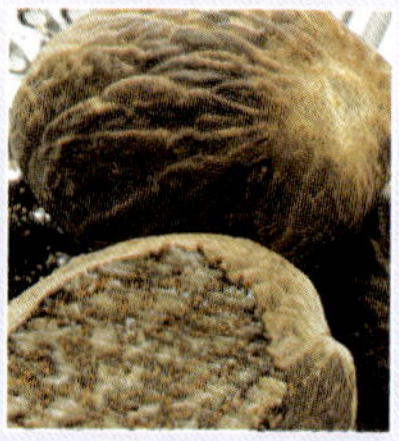

# lemon *Citrus limonum*

Lemon essential oil has a zesty, fruity sharp fragrance, with sweet and sherbet-like notes as it evaporates. It fills the air with a fresh and bright aroma, and is immediately enlivening to the senses.

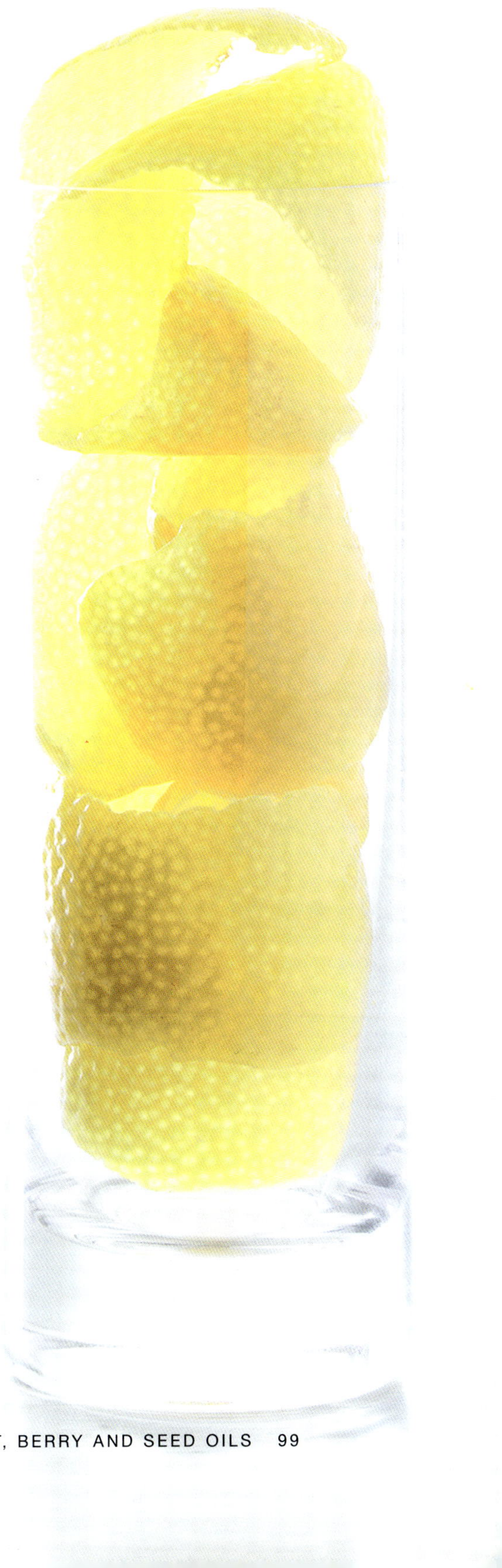

### Botanical source and background

Lemon is a member of the Rutaceae family of citrus fruit trees. Its oil is produced in Italy, Sicily, Florida and California. An evergreen growing to 20ft (6m) tall, the lemon tree has pointed shiny leaves and fragrant flowers that turn into the yellow fruit. An average tree will produce a thousand lemons in a good year. Citrus fruit originated in China, and the lemon was possibly brought to southern Europe via Persia and the Middle East as early as the second century. The word "lemon" comes from the Arabic *limun*. Citrus trees were taken to the West Indies for cultivation in the 15th century and have thrived there ever since. Lemon essential oil is used commercially for flavouring confectionary, and lemon juice has been used traditionally to lighten the hair and the skin.

### Extraction and storage

Lemon essential oil is expressed from the fruit's peel (see p.19); around a thousand lemons will yield is about 1lb (650g) oil. In the refrigerator lemon oil has a maximum shelf life of one year; and at cool room temperature (54°F/12°C) just six months. Buy it in small amounts and use it fresh: old oil turns cloudy and loses its fragrance.

### Physical and psychological effects

*Circulatory tonic:* tones and improves the circulation
*Diuretic:* tones the kidneys and lymphatic system in detoxifying or anti-cellulite treatments
*Astringent:* tones large, open pores on the face, balances greasy skin and improves the appearance of any visible thread or broken veins
*Antidepressant:* lifts depression, low spirits, lack of confidence and anxiety

### Special lemon blends, in 4tsp (20ml) carrier oil

*Anti-cellulite*: Lemon 4 drops, Cypress 2 drops, Juniper 4 drops
*Oily/combination face tonic:* Lemon 1 drop, Frankincense 2 drops, Geranium 2 drops
*Mental-rejuvenator:* Lemon 4 drops, Rosemary 4 drops, Peppermint 2 drops

### Safety information

Lemon oil is phototoxic; if you massage a lemon blend onto the skin, do not expose the skin to strong sunlight or a sunbed for 12 hours following application.

# mandarin *Citrus reticulata*

Mandarin essential oil has a bitter-sweet aroma – green and piercing, with sweeter notes as it evaporates. It is pungent, and full of zest and brightness, instantly perfuming the air with uplifting citrus freshness.

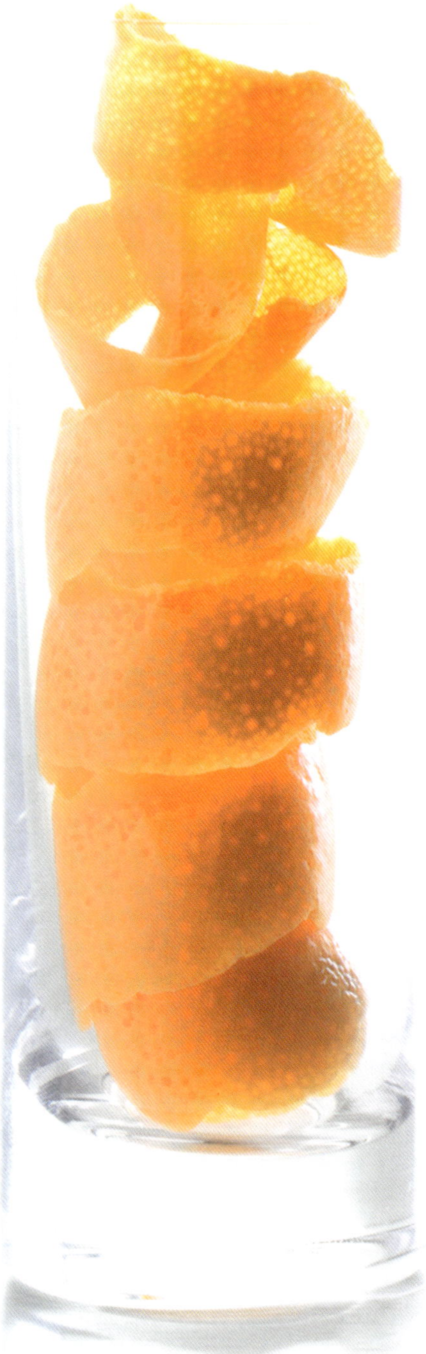

### Botanical source and background

Mandarin belongs to the Rutaceae family, originally native to China and the Far East. It is commercially cultivated in Italy, Spain, Cyprus and the Middle East. The tangerine is the same species, but is the name given to fruit grown in Texas, Florida and California. It is a small evergreen tree that grows up to 20ft (6m) tall and has glossy, dark green leaves, white flowers and small orange fruit with a shiny rind. In ancient China, these fruit were given as gifts to the rulers, the Mandarins, and were named after them. The trees were successfully introduced to southern Europe in the 18th century. Because they were available in winter, they became part of Christmas celebrations; the small fragrant fruit were regarded as special stocking-fillers. Today the flavour and fragrance industries use mandarin essential oil extensively in confectionary, drinks, toiletry products and soaps.

### Extraction and storage

Mandarin essential oil is a golden yellow colour and is extracted by expression. It will last up to a year in the refrigerator, or six months at cool room temperature (54°F/12°C). Buy small quantities and use it fresh: it will smell rancid and turn cloudy as it ages.

### Physical and psychological effects

*Digestive tonic:* stimulates the digestion, and eases cramps and wind
*Liver tonic:* stimulates the liver to break down fats
*Skin-toning:* tones open pores and cleanses skin; good for greasy or acne-prone skin
*Antidepressant:* uplifts moods, especially the emotional swings associated with PMS
*Mentally-refreshing:* eases mental fatigue

### Special mandarin blends, in 4tsp (20ml) carrier oil

*Facial blemish tonic:* Mandarin 2 drops, Cypress 1 drop, Lavender 2 drops
*Pre-menstrual mood-enhancer:* Mandarin 4 drops, Neroli 2 drops, Geranium 4 drops
*Mental-rejuvenator:* Mandarin 4 drops, Myrtle 4 drops, Spanish sage 2 drops
*Child's tummy soother:* Mandarin 2 drops, Roman chamomile 2 drops, Lavender 1 drop

### Safety information

Mandarin is not regarded as phototoxic and is very mild and safe to use.

# sweet orange *Citrus sinensis*

Sweet orange essential oil has a light, citrusy aroma – fresh and gently tangy, becoming softer as it evaporates. A highly attractive and mouth-watering fragrance, it is full of fruity sweetness.

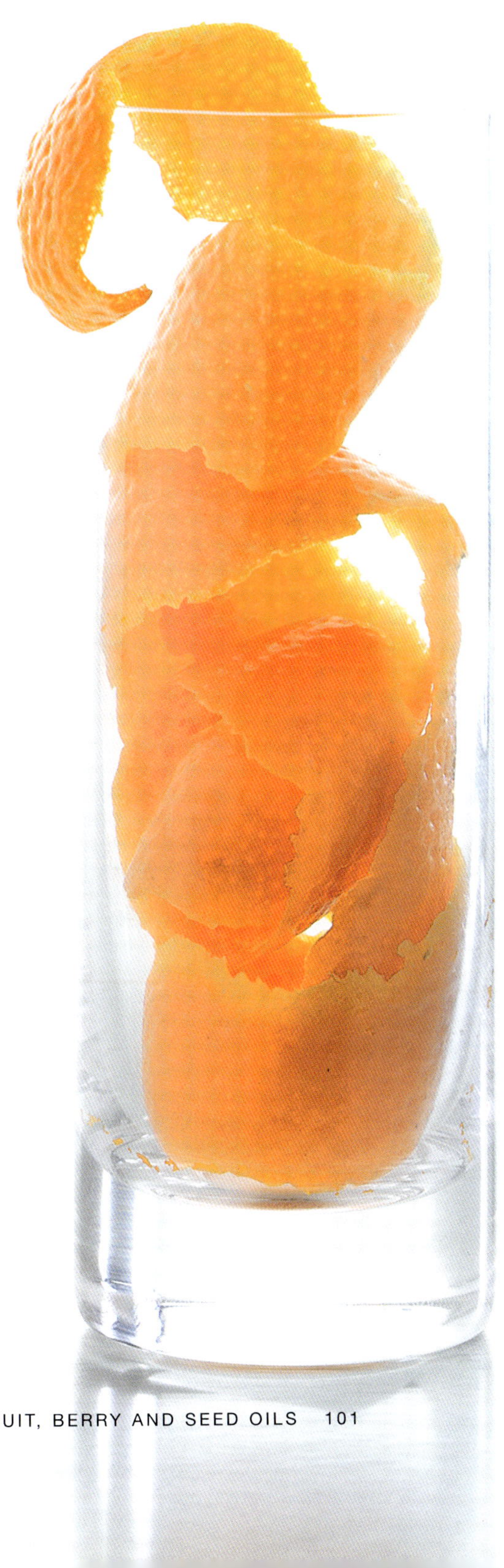

### Botanical source and background

Sweet orange is another member of the Rutaceae family of citrus trees, originally native to China. It is eaten as a dessert fruit and is grown commercially on a large scale in Brazil, Florida and Israel. The sweet orange tree grows to around 24ft (8m) in height. It is evergreen, with soft, rich green leaves, white flowers and attractive orange fruit with a smooth rind. The early Arabs were the first to write about the orange, and the word itself comes from the Arabic *naranj*. The exact date of its arrival in Europe is not known, but it was successfully introduced from Europe to the West Indies in the 15th century, and from there to the Americas. Sweet orange essential oil is widely used as a food flavouring in confectionary and also as a fragrance note in soaps and toiletry products.

### Extraction and storage

Sweet orange essential oil is extracted by expression (see p.19). It will keep only up to one year in the refrigerator and just six months at cool room temperature (54°F/12°C); old oil turns cloudy and smells sour.

### Physical and psychological effects

*Antispasmodic:* calms stomach aches or cramps, particularly in children
*Mildly diuretic:* stimulates the kidneys to detoxify the system
*Skin-soothing:* calms irritation, gently rejuvenates tired, lacklustre skin
*Nervous sedative:* soothes and calms anxiety, emotional upset and irritability
*Antidepressant:* improves mood, immediately cheers the spirits

### Special sweet orange blends, in 4tsp (20ml) carrier oil

*Child's tummy settler (ages 3 to 10):* Sweet orange 2 drops, Roman chamomile 2 drops
*Facial skin treat:* Sweet orange 2 drops, Palmarosa 2 drops, Rosewood 1 drop
*Mental-soother:* Sweet orange 4 drops, Sandalwood 4 drops, Carrot seed 2 drops
*Mood-enhancer:* Sweet orange 4 drops, Rose otto 2 drops, Frankincense 4 drops

### Safety information

Sweet orange is the mildest of the citrus oils, and is not regarded as phototoxic. It is non-irritating and non-sensitizing and a useful essential oil for children.

# grapefruit *Citrus x paradisi*

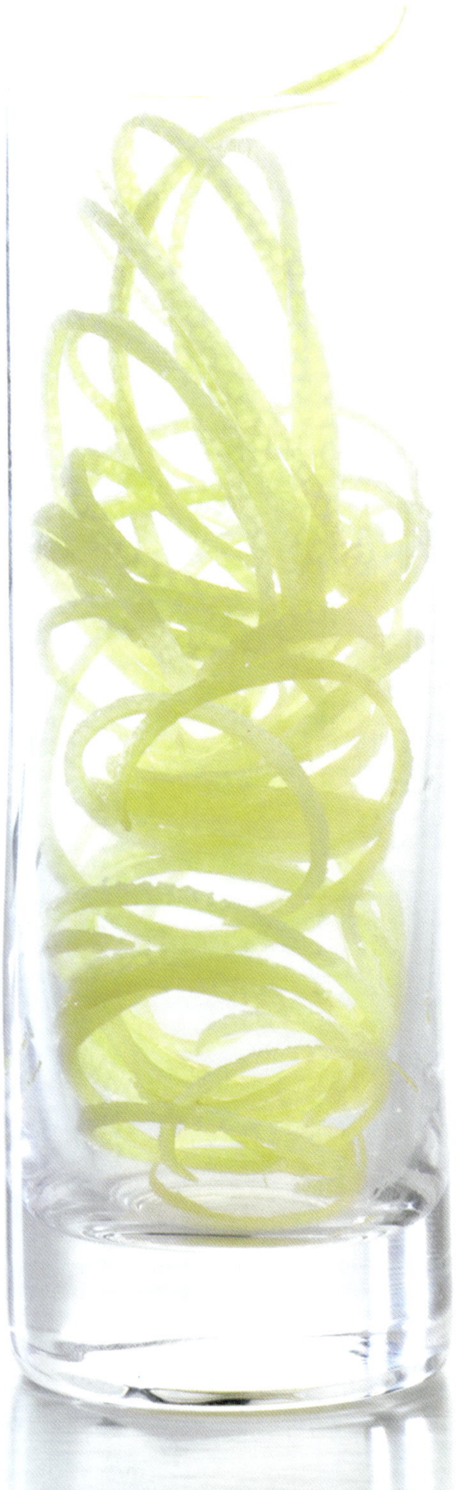

Grapefruit has the most bitter-sweet aroma of all the citrus fruits, but it is also extremely zesty and bright, full of sharp freshness with an underlying sweetness. It is stimulating to the senses and uplifting to the mind.

## Botanical source and background

Grapefruit belongs to the Rutaceae family, and its essential oil is produced mainly in Brazil, Florida and Israel. Grapefruit trees are evergreen and grow up to 30ft (10m) tall. They have glossy green leaves, star-shaped white aromatic flowers and large round fruit with shiny yellow peel. The precise origin of the grapefruit is a mystery; it is a hybrid, and one of its parents, the pumello fruit, was originally brought to Europe by early medieval Arab traders. It is likely that the pumello cross-pollinated itself with the sweet orange when both species were introduced to the West Indies, and so created the grapefruit. Grapefruit oil is used as a food and drink flavouring, and in natural cosmetics. It detoxifies the body and has become a favourite in aromatherapy spa treatments to improve lymphatic drainage.

## Extraction and storage

Grapefruit essential oil is expressed, or squeezed, from the peel of the fruit. It will keep for up to one year in the refrigerator, or six months at cool room temperature (54°F/12°C). It is best to buy the oil in small amounts and use it fresh.

## Physical and psychological effects

*Diuretic:* detoxifies the system, helps tone up areas of cellulite
*Skin-toning:* tones and cleanses oily or combination skin
*Immune-boosting:* assists convalescence after immune infections
*Antidepressant:* transforms negative feelings and improves self-confidence
*Mentally-rejuvenating:* improves mental function and concentration

## Special grapefruit blends, in 4tsp (20ml) carrier oil

*Oily-skin tonic:* Grapefruit 2 drops, Tea tree 1 drop, Atlas cedarwood 2 drops
*Anti-cellulite:* Grapefruit 4 drops, Fennel 4 drops, Juniper berry 2 drops
*Immune tonic:* Grapefruit 4 drops, Cardamom 2 drops, Ginger 4 drops
*Mental-booster:* Grapefruit 4 drops, Rosemary 4 drops, Spanish sage 2 drops

## Safety information

Grapefruit essential oil is phototoxic: if you massage a blend containing it into the skin, do not expose the skin to strong sunlight or a sunbed for 12 hours following application.

# coriander seed *Coriandrum sativum*

Coriander seed essential oil is warm, spicy and sweet, with underlying hints of musk and fruitiness. Its pleasant fragrance is literally mouth-watering, as it stimulates the body's digestive juices.

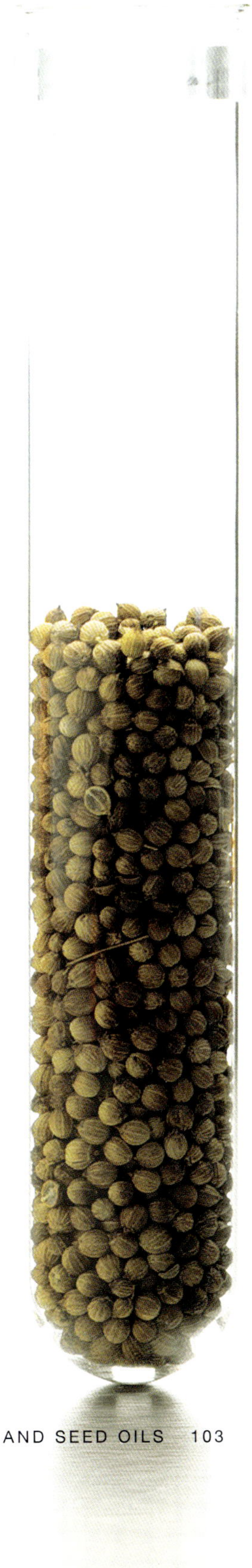

### Botanical source and background

A member of the vast Umbelliferae plant family, coriander was originally native to the eastern Mediterranean before it spread over southern Europe. Today the US, Russia, Serbia, Croatia and Romania produce it as a herb, dried spice and essential oil. Coriander is an annual plant growing up to 3ft (1m) tall, with branching stems and fresh green leaves with toothed edges. Its tiny white flowers form in umbels (clusters of stalks resembling an upturned umbrella). Brown seeds follow, which fall as soon as they are ripe. The whole plant has a highly pungent aroma. Coriander was known to Ancient Greek physicians, and, in the 1st century CE, Roman writer Pliny mentions its popularity in Ancient Egypt, where it is still widely used in cookery and medicine today. Indian cookery and Ayurvedic medicine also use the herb and its seeds as a digestive tonic.

### Extraction and storage

Steam distillation of the crushed ripe seeds produces a colourless essential oil, which will keep for up to two years in the refrigerator, and one year at cool room temperature (54°F/12°C).

### Physical and psychological effects

*Detoxifying:* cleanses the kidneys and the lymphatic system, removes excess toxins
*Digestive tonic:* stimulates the digestive juices, improves liver function
*Antispasmodic:* calms stomach aches and spasms, constipation or nervous diarrhea
*Immune-boosting:* fortifies the body against viral or bacterial infections
*Nervous restorative:* helps overcome insomnia, nervous tension and anxiety

### Special coriander seed blends, in 4tsp (20ml) carrier oil

*Detoxifier:* Coriander seed 4 drops, Fennel 4 drops, Juniper berry 2 drops
*Digestive tonic:* Coriander seed 4 drops, Nutmeg 2 drops, Sweet orange 4 drops
*Immune tonic:* Coriander seed 4 drops, Cardamom 4 drops, Black pepper 2 drops
*Nerve-soother:* Coriander seed 4 drops, Neroli 2 drops, Sandalwood 4 drops

### Safety information

Coriander seed essential oil is non-toxic, non-irritating and non-sensitizing.

# cumin seed *Cuminum cyminum*

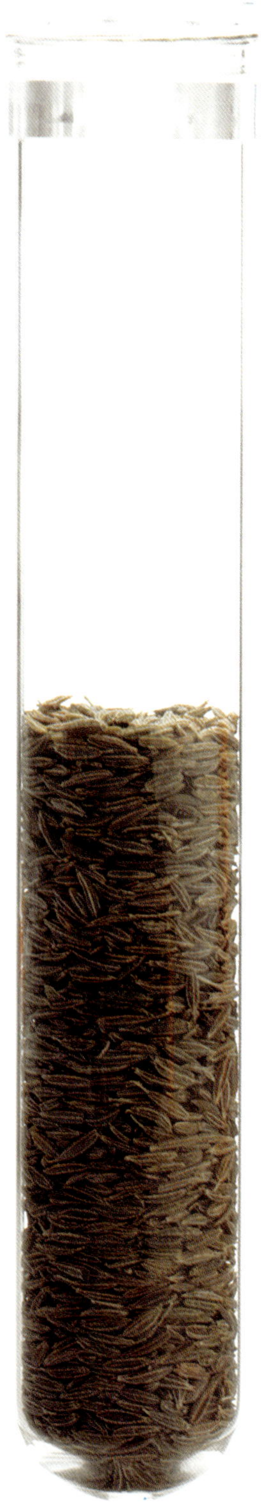

Cumin seed oil has a deeply spicy and musky aroma, becoming warmer and richer as it evaporates. It is an unusual fragrance full of exotic notes, creating a sense of faraway places.

## Botanical source and background

Cumin belongs to the vast Umbelliferae plant family. Originally cultivated in the Far East, it is now commercially produced in India, Spain and France. It is a small annual herb, up to 2ft (60cm) tall, with slender stems and feathery leaves. Small pinkish-white flowers form in clusters in early summer, and become highly aromatic seeds. Cumin has been used as a medicine and a spice for millennia. It is mentioned in the Bible, as well as in the works of Ancient Greek physicians such as Hippocrates and Dioscorides. In the 1st century CE, the Roman writer Pliny tells that the ancients ate ground cumin seed in bread for its digestive medicinal properties. In medieval Europe it was a popular culinary flavouring in savoury and sweet dishes. Cumin is found in many Indian spice blends, and is a staple of Ayurvedic medicine, used as an immune tonic and a digestive remedy. Cumin seed oil is found in food and drink flavourings, and is also used as a warm fragrance note in perfumery.

## Extraction and storage

Steam distillation of cumin seeds yields a very pale yellow essential oil, which will last up to two years in the refrigerator, and one year at cool room temperature (54°F/12°C).

## Physical and psychological effects

*Antispasmodic:* soothes stomach cramps and regulates bowel rhythm
*Immune-boosting:* helps fight bacterial and viral infections; eases respiratory problems
*Circulatory tonic:* helps poor circulation especially in hands and feet
*Nervous sedative:* comforts and soothes the mind

## Special cumin seed blends, in 4tsp (20ml) carrier oil

*Stomach-soother:* Cumin seed 2 drops, Coriander seed 4 drops, Roman chamomile 4 drops
*Immune tonic:* Cumin seed 2 drops, Sandalwood 4 drops, Cardamom 4 drops
*Circulation tonic:* Cumin seed 2 drops, Ginger 4 drops, Lemon 4 drops
*Nerve-soother:* Cumin seed 2 drops, May chang 4 drops, Lavender 4 drops

## Safety information

Cumin seed essential oil is phototoxic: if you massage a blend containing it into the skin, do not expose the skin to strong sunlight or a sunbed for 12 hours following application.

# carrot seed *Daucus carota*

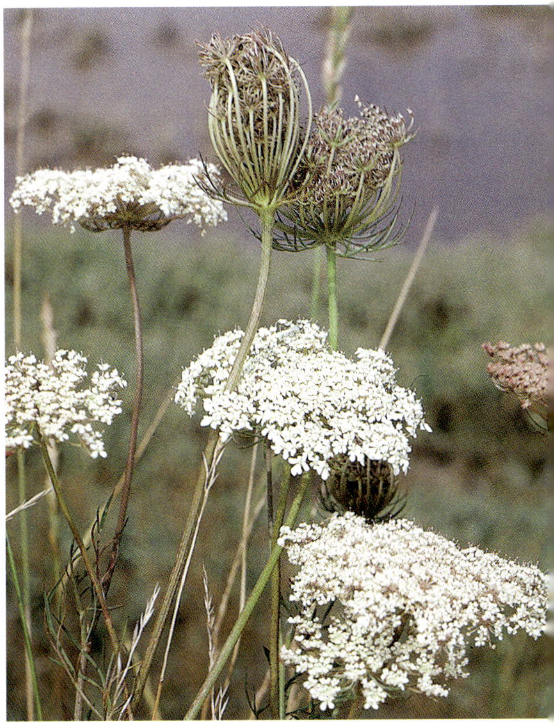

Carrot seed essential oil has an unusual aroma – warm, earthy and woody, with sweet and slightly dry undertones. It is instantly calming and soothing to the body and mind, and is even subtly spicy as it evaporates.

### Botanical source and background

Another member of the extensive Umbelliferae family, the carrot is native to Asia, Europe and North Africa and was introduced to North America. Most carrot seed essential oil is produced in France. The plant is an annual, up to 5ft (1.5m) tall, with feathery leaves, flat-topped clusters of tiny white flowers and small aromatic seeds. The cultivated form of *Daucus carota* produces the familiar orange root which is eaten as a vegetable. The essential oil is from the seeds of the original wild species, which has a small white root with a much stronger taste. The wild carrot was well-known to the Ancient Greeks who enjoyed its pungent flavour. It was first called *carota* in the writings of Roman cookery enthusiast Apicius Caelius, in 230 CE. The botanical name *daucus* is from the Greek *dais*, meaning "to burn", a reference to the pungent taste of the root. Carrots were used in traditional Western herbal medicine as diuretics and digestives.

### Extraction and storage

Steam distillation of ripe carrot seeds produces a yellowish essential oil, which will last up to two years in the refrigerator, and one year at cool room temperature (54°F/12°C).

### Physical and psychological effects

*Liver tonic:* stimulates the liver and assists its healthy function
*Detoxifying:* tones the kidneys and lymphatic system; useful in anti-cellulite massage
*Antispasmodic:* eases menstrual pain and stomach cramps
*Skin-rejuvenator:* improves mature, dry or environmentally damaged skin
*Nervous restorative:* helps relieve insomnia, nervous tension, anxiety and restlessness

### Special carrot seed blends, in 4tsp (20ml) carrier oil

*Liver tonic:* Carrot seed 4 drops, Grapefruit 4 drops, Fennel 2 drops
*Menstrual-soother:* Carrot seed 4 drops, Sweet marjoram 4 drops, Vetiver 2 drops
*Facial skin tonic:* Carrot seed 2 drops, Neroli 1 drop, Frankincense 2 drops
*Nerve-soother:* Carrot seed 4 drops, Ylang ylang 2 drops, Rosewood 4 drops

### Safety information

Carrot seed essential oil is non-toxic, non-irritating and non-sensitizing.

# cardamom *Elettaria cardamomum*

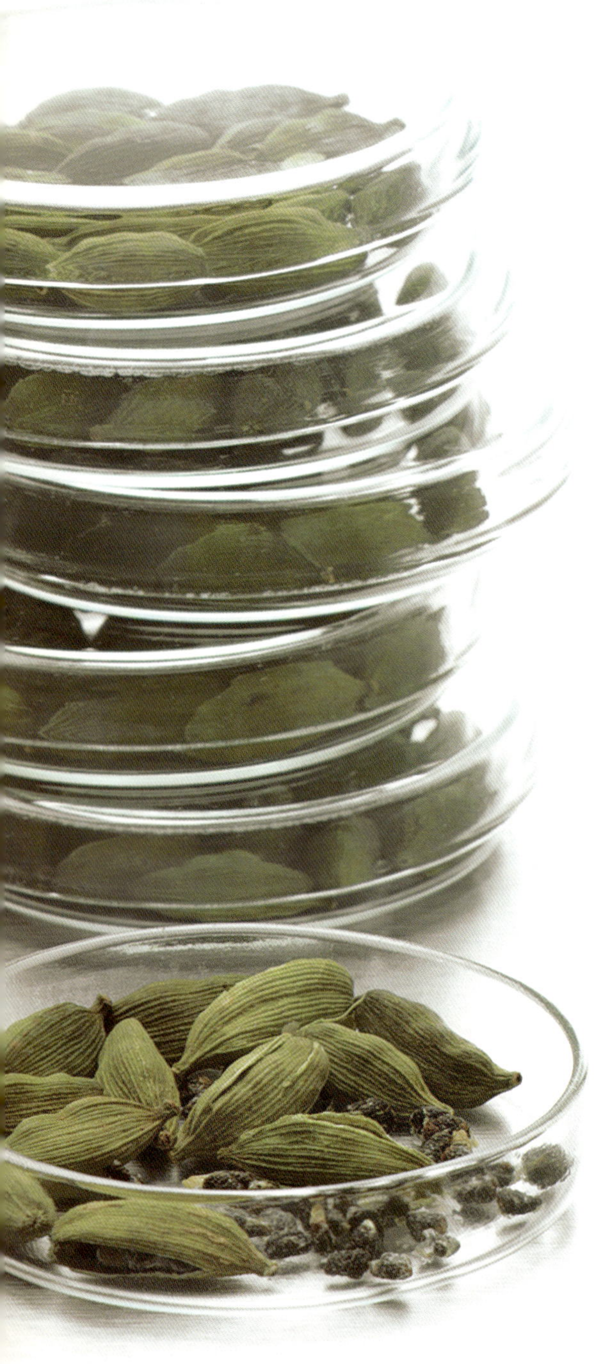

Cardamom essential oil has a warm, rich and fruity aroma with soft and woody undertones, becoming softer and spicier as it evaporates. It has an immediately cheering and uplifting effect on the mind.

### Botanical source and background

Cardamom is a member of the plant family Zingiberaceae, which includes other spices such as ginger. Native to tropical Asia, it is now commercially cultivated in India, Sri Lanka and Guatemala. Cardamom has tall slender stalks with pairs of large, lance-shaped leaves arranged symmetrically, and can grow up to 12ft (4m) in height. It produces small whitish-yellow flowers, which turn into hard seed pods containing tiny black, shiny, aromatic seeds. Cardamom is a key ingredient in Far Eastern cookery and traditional medicine. It has been used in India and China for at least 3,000 years to treat respiratory and immune problems, digestive imbalances, and urinary infections, as well as to flavour sweet and savoury dishes. The Ancient Egyptians used cardamom seeds in incense and perfumery, and in medicinal ointments, and Ancient Greek physicians used cardamom to treat coughs and stomach pains. The botanical name *Elettaria* derives from the Hindu name for the plant. In the East, the pods and seeds are chewed to sweeten the breath.

### Extraction and storage

Steam distillation of the seeds produces a pale, almost colourless essential oil, which will last up to two years in the refrigerator, or one year at cool room temperature (54°F/12°C).

### Physical and psychological effects

*Digestive tonic:* tones up digestion, regulates bowel rhythm and relieves constipation
*Expectorant:* helps chesty or tight coughs and other respiratory infections
*Immune-boosting:* a superb immune-booster for preventive massage treatments.
*Antidepressant:* uplifts negative feelings and transforms low spirits

### Special cardamom blends, in 4tsp (20ml) carrier oil

*Digestive tonic:* Cardamom 4 drops, Black pepper 4 drops, Peppermint 2 drops
*Respiratory tonic:* Cardamom 4 drops, Atlas cedarwood 4 drops, Nutmeg 2 drops
*Immune tonic:* Cardamom 4 drops, Ginger 2 drops, Myrtle 4 drops
*Nervous tonic:* Cardamom 4 drops, Sweet orange 4 drops, Ylang ylang 2 drops

### Safety information

Cardamom essential oil is non-toxic, non-irritating and non-sensitizing.

# fennel *Foeniculum vulgare var. dulce*

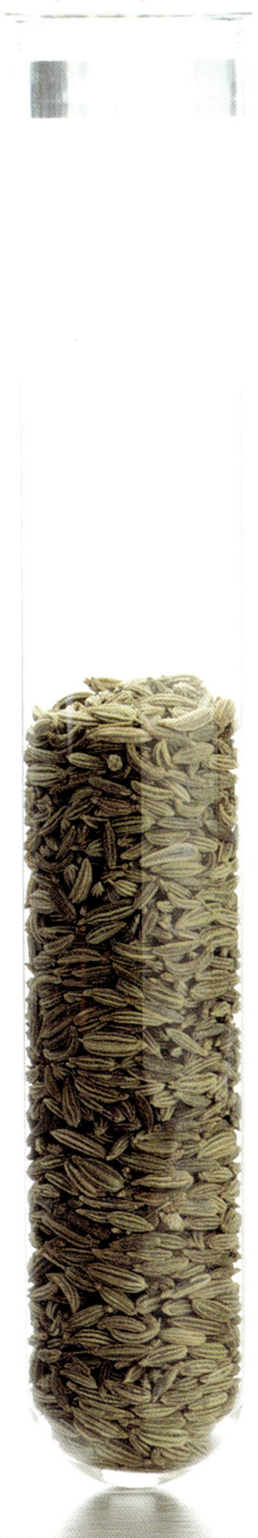

Fennel essential oil has a powerful aniseed-like fragrance – fresh and tenacious, with sweet, spicy and peppery undertones. It instantly uplifts the mind and fortifies the spirits with its refreshing pungency.

### Botanical source and background

Fennel is one of the best-known members of the Umbelliferae family. Extensively cultivated worldwide, it's oil is produced in Spain, France, Hungary, Germany, Italy and Greece. Fennel is a tall biennial herb growing up to 6ft (2m), with stout stems and wide branches. It produces finely branched, golden-green leaves, and large, flat clusters of yellow flowers. Its slightly curved seeds are grey-green in colour with a pleasant taste. Fennel's Latin name *Foeniculum* means "like hay", because of its odour. In the 1st century CE, Pliny mentioned at least 22 medicinal uses for fennel, and it was a popular ingredient in Roman meat sauces. The Anglo-Saxons also used it in cooking and in medicine. The 17th-century English herbalist Culpeper used fennel to treat a range of digestive complaints.

### Extraction and storage

Steam distillation of fennel seeds produces a colourless essential oil, which will last up to two years in the refrigerator, and one year at cool room temperature (54°F/12°C).

### Physical and psychological effects

*Diuretic:* tones the kidneys, encouraging loss of excess fluid
*Hormone-regulating:* balances the menstrual cycle and eases PMS
*Skin-toning:* deep-cleanses pores and dissolves excess oil; rejuvenates mature skin
*Antispasmodic:* eases stomach cramps, indigestion and nausea
*Mentally-rejuvenating:* helps concentration and uplifts mental stress

### Special fennel blends, in 4tsp (20ml) carrier oil

*Detoxifier:* Fennel 2 drops, Grapefruit 4 drops, Cypress 4 drops
*Hormone-balancer:* Fennel 2 drops, Geranium 4 drops, May chang 4 drops
*Mature-skin tonic:* Fennel 1 drop, Rose otto 1 drop, Sandalwood 3 drops
*Digestive tonic:* Fennel 2 drops, Peppermint 2 drops, Sweet orange 6 drops
*Mental-refresher:* Fennel 2 drops, Rosemary 4 drops, Eucalyptus 4 drops

### Safety information

Fennel oil is not advised during pregnancy or for babies or infants. Take care never to exceed the stated number of drops in a blend, and do not use on people with epilepsy.

# juniper berry *Juniperus communis*

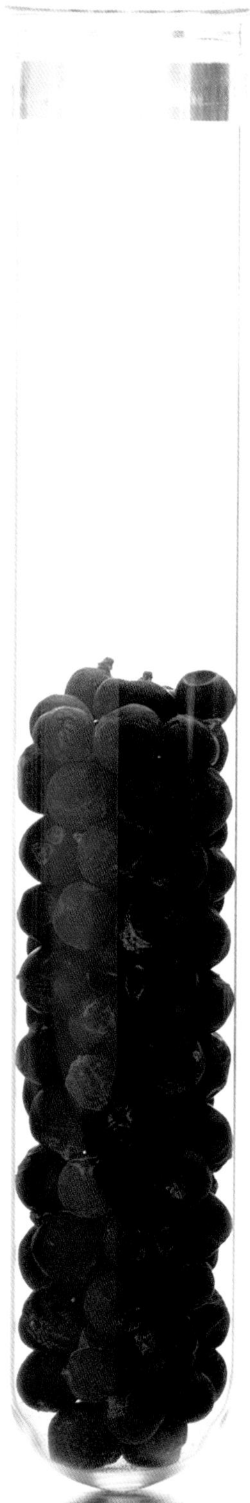

Juniper essential oil has a fresh, green pungent aroma with underlying woody, peppery notes, becoming softer and sweeter as it evaporates. It has a stimulating and fresh aroma, and clears the air.

## Botanical source and background

Juniper belongs to the Cupressaceae family, which includes many evergreen shrubs and trees. Its oil is produced in Italy, Austria, Hungary, Serbia and Croatia. This prickly shrub has green berries which take up to two years to ripen to a black colour, when they contain the maximum essential oil. Juniper was used by the Ancient Egyptians in the mummification process, and was burned in Ancient Greece as an air purifier. Western herbal medicine regards juniper as a potent detoxifying remedy. Juniper berries are a key flavouring in gin, and in Central Europe juniper preserve is eaten in winter as an immune tonic.

## Extraction and storage

Steam distillation of ripe juniper berries yields a colourless essential oil. Ripe juniper berry oil is the best quality; oil from unripe berries and twigs has an inferior odour and lower therapeutic effect. Juniper berry oil will keep for up to two years in the refrigerator, or up to one year at cool room temperature (54°F/12°C).

## Physical and psychological effects

*Circulatory tonic:* warms cold hands and feet, and chilly limbs
*Diuretic:* detoxifies the system, removing excess fluid
*Skin-toning:* dissolves excess skin oils and tones large open pores
*Mentally-refreshing:* improves poor concentration and eases mental fatigue
*Emotionally-cleansing:* cleanses the mind of negativity and assists clear thinking

## Special juniper blends, in 4tsp (20ml) carrier oil

*Muscle and circulation tonic:* Juniper berry 4 drops, Scotch pine 2 drops, Myrtle 4 drops
*Oily-skin tonic:* Juniper berry 1 drop, Cypress 2 drops, Petitgrain 2 drops
*Mental-rejuvenator:* Juniper berry 2 drops, Rosemary 4 drops, Lavendin 4 drops
*Emotional-cleanser:* Juniper berry 2 drops, Spanish sage 4 drops, Lemon 4 drops

## Safety information

Juniper berry essential oil has a powerful tonic effect on the uterus, so its use is not advised during pregnancy. Also, it is not recommended for those with highly allergy-prone skin. Otherwise the oil is non-irritating and non-toxic.

# may chang *Litsea cubeba*

May chang essential oil has a pronouced lemon-sherbet aroma, full of fizzy, citrusy notes. It evaporates to become sweet and soft and is totally different in aroma and effect to lemon oil (see p.99).

## Botanical source and background

May chang belongs to the Lauraceae family which includes many aromatic trees. It is native to China, which produces most of the essential oil on the world market. A small tropical tree, it has delicate branches and finely textured, soft leaves with a lemony fragrance. A relative newcomer to the aromatherapist's kit, may chang has excited interest thanks to Chinese research highlighting its ability to calm erratic heartbeat patterns. May chang essential oil is similar in composition to lemongrass oil, but has a much gentler effect and is easier to blend successfully. In Traditional Chinese Medicine, may chang is used to treat chills, fevers, headaches, muscular aches and chronic respiratory problems such as asthma. The fragrance industry uses may chang oil extensively in toiletries and perfumes. It is also used as a natural flavouring in confectionary.

## Extraction and storage

Steam distillation of may chang fruit yields a pale yellow essential oil, which will last up to two years in the refrigerator, or one year at cool room temperature (54°F/12°C).

## Physical and psychological effects

*Respiratory tonic:* assists breathing problems or asthma
*Heart tonic:* benefits the heart, regulates irregular heartbeat
*Skin-toning:* tones oily or combination skin, tightens pores
*Nervous restorative:* clears the head, refreshing the mind

## Special may chang blends, in 4tsp (20ml) carrier oil

*Respiratory support:* May chang 2 drops, Atlas cedarwood 4 drops, Myrrh 4 drops
*Heart-soother:* May chang 2 drops, Rose otto 2 drops, Sweet orange 6 drops
*Oily-skin tonic:* May chang 1 drop, Lavender 2 drops, Myrtle 2 drops
*Mental-rejuvenator:* May chang 2 drops, Petitgrain 4 drops, Lavendin 4 drops

## Safety information

Although may chang is milder than lemongrass, it still contains a high percentage of powerful constituents called aldehydes. It is not recommended for use on sensitive, allergy-prone skin, children below the age of 10, or individuals with eczema.

# nutmeg *Myristica fragrans*

Nutmeg essential oil has a rich, spicy, sweet fragrance with fruity and woody undertones, and a deep softness as it evaporates. It instantly uplifts and cheers the spirit and has strong associations with Christmas.

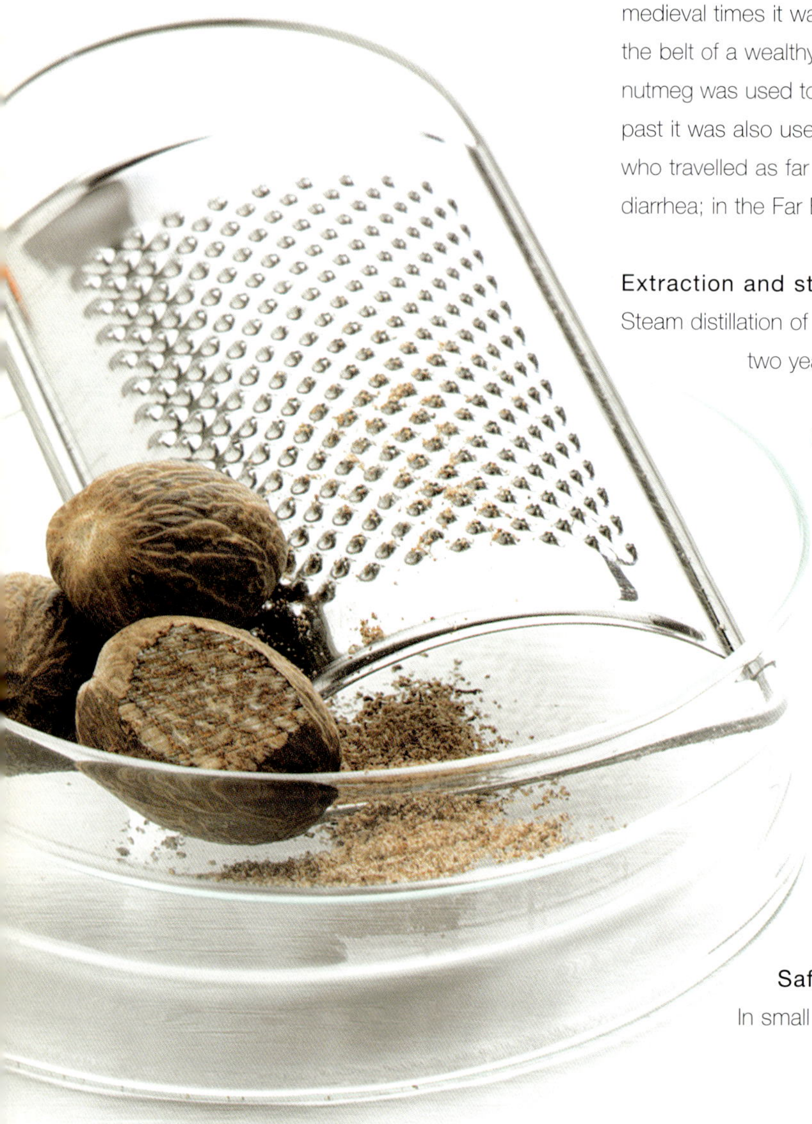

### Botanical source and background

Nutmeg belongs to the plant family Myristicaceae, and is extensively cultivated in Indonesia, Sri Lanka and Grenada. An evergreen tree, it grows up to 60ft (20m) and has dark leaves and yellow flowers which become the fruit. This fruit is dried before being sold as a spice or processed for essential oil. Nutmeg has been used for centuries as a domestic spice; in medieval times it was considered so valuable that it was often worn locked in a small box at the belt of a wealthy housewife. In the 14th century, a drink of hot milk sprinkled with ground nutmeg was used to help insomnia. Nutmeg is a favourite flavouring in sweet dishes but in the past it was also used to flavour to meat. It probably came to Europe with early Arab traders who travelled as far as India. Western herbal medicine uses nutmeg to treat indigestion and diarrhea; in the Far East the oil is used to treat muscular aches and rheumatism.

### Extraction and storage

Steam distillation of dried nutmeg yields a colourless essential oil, which will keep for up to two years in the refrigerator, and one year at cool room temperature (54°F/12°C).

### Physical and psychological effects

*Digestive tonic:* stimulates the digestion
*Circulatory tonic:* warms the circulation; helps stiff, aching muscles
*Immune-boosting:* builds resistance to bacterial or viral infections
*Antidepressant:* uplifts negative thinking, alleviates mental pressure

### Special nutmeg blends, in 4tsp (20ml) carrier oil

*Digestive tonic:* Nutmeg 2 drops, Ginger 4 drops, May chang 4 drops
*Circulation-booster:* Nutmeg 2 drops, Cardamon 4 drops, Black pepper 4 drops
*Immune tonic:* Nutmeg 2 drops, Manuka 4 drops, Lemon 4 drops
*Mental-rejuvenator:* Nutmeg 2 drops, Mandarin 4 drops, Atlas cedarwood 4 drops

### Safety information

In small amounts nutmeg oil is non-toxic, non-irritating and non-sensitizing.

# black pepper *Piper nigrum*

Black pepper essential oil has a warm, pungent, spicy aroma with dry and woody undertones and a slight sweetness on evaporation. It has a penetrating fragrance that is bracing and powerful.

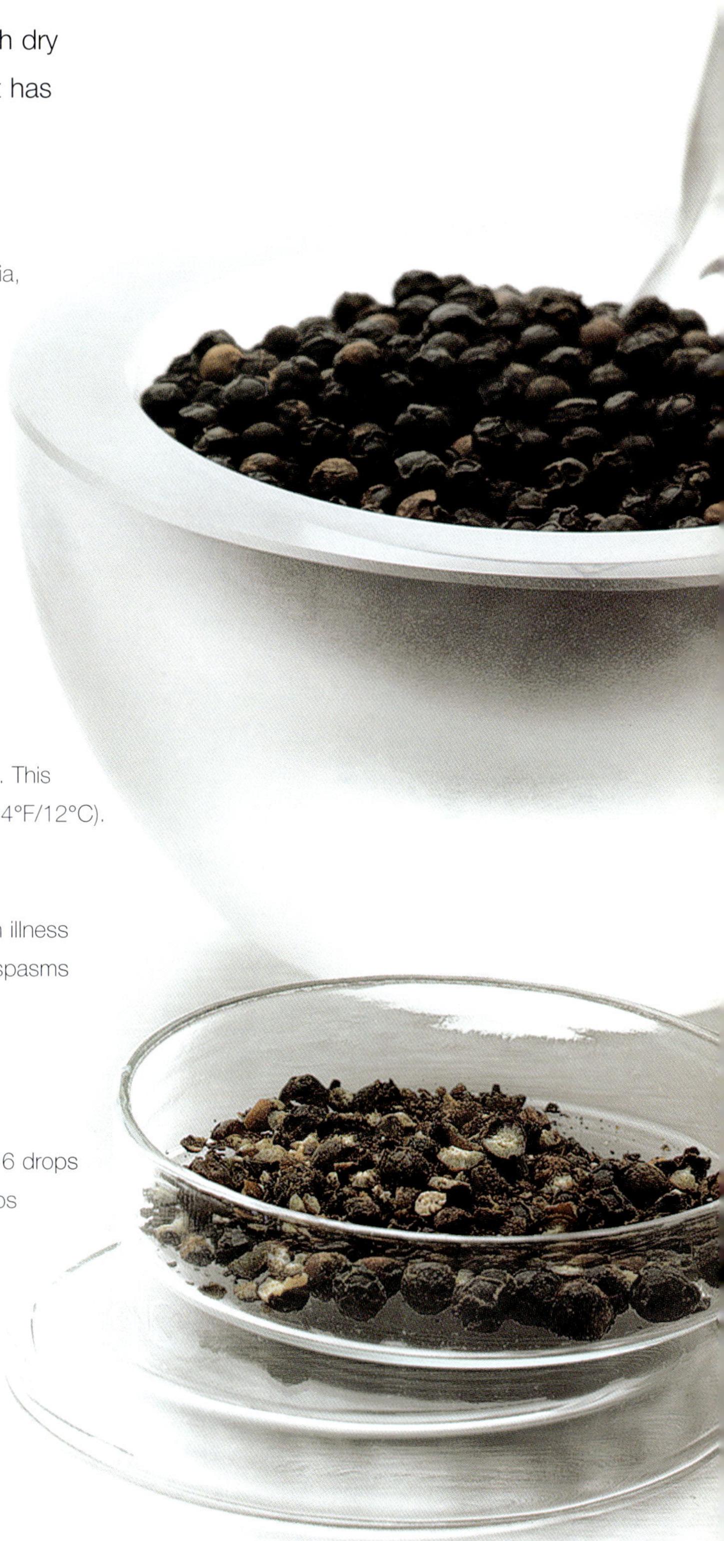

### Botanical source and background

A member of the Piperaceae family, black pepper is produced in India, Malaysia, Indonesia, Masagascar and China for use as a spice and an essential oil. It comes from a vigorous climbing plant, with heart-shaped, dark green leaves, that produces long clusters of flowers which turn into tiny round fruit – the peppercorns. These are picked and dried in the sun. Black peppercorns come from the dried unripe fruit; white pepper is produced from the dried ripe fruit with the rind removed. Black peppercorns have been used for more than 4,000 years in cooking and medicine in the Far East, particularly in China and India where digestive, immune and circulatory problems are still treated with the berries. The spice was once considered so valuable that Attila the Hun demanded 3000lb (1360kg) of peppercorns as a ransom for the city of Rome.

### Extraction and storage

Steam distillation of dried crushed peppercorns yields a colourless essential oil. This lasts up to two years in the refrigerator, or one year at cool room temperature (54°F/12°C).

### Physical and psychological effects

*Appetite stimulant:* encourages appetite, especially during convalescence from illness
*Antispasmodic:* eases constipation, sluggish digestion, stomach cramps and spasms
*Circulatory tonic:* warms the circulation; eases aches, pains and stiffness
*Immune-boosting:* fortifies the system against viral and bacterial infections

### Special black pepper blends, in 4tsp (20ml) carrier oil

*Appetite-reviver:* Black pepper 2 drops, Lemongrass 2 drops, Coriander seed 6 drops
*Circulation tonic:* Black pepper 2 drops, Rosemary 4 drops, Eucalyptus 4 drops
*Immune tonic:* Black pepper 2 drops, Cardamom 4 drops, Lemon 4 drops

### Safety information

Black pepper has a reddening effect on the skin because it stimulates local circulation: it is not recommended for highly sensitive or delicate skins. Otherwise the oil is non-toxic.

# wood, resin and gum oils

This is a fascinating group of essential oils, with aromatic ingredients that have links far back to the ancient history of perfumery, ritual and medicine.The oils all originate in exotic locations, and have connections with cultures and philosophies that are thousands of years old. Their protective and healing properties are still relevant today.

Some commentators believe that humans have evolved a special relationship with these particular woods, resins and gums because they contain ingredients that mimic aspects of our own odour – in other words we gravitated toward these trees in times past because in some ways they smelled like we do! Musky, woody and sweet notes in these fragrances became the fixatives, or base notes, in ancient fragrance compounds. Burned as incense, these aromas were hugely evocative to ancient peoples; the Egyptians had a hieroglyph for perfume that showed smoke rising from an altar where incense burned.

Botanists explain the presence of aromatic compounds in these trees and shrubs as having a protective purpose. The aroma and taste of essential oils in wood is believed to discourage insects that try to bore holes into the bark to lay eggs, an activity that could be potentially damaging to the tree. Aromatic compounds containing essential oils are found in the heartwood of branches and trunks, which is also the part of the tree that transports water and nutrients around it; by protecting these pathways from insects, the tree can grow safely to its full height and spread.

The Ancient Egyptians understood the potential of aromatic woods and made good use of them – the red heartwood of the atlas cedarwood tree was used for making coffins, furniture and sacred objects for royal tombs. Thousands of years later when tombs were opened, these objects were remarkably preserved, thanks to the essential oil which kept gnawing insects away. Amazingly, many of these objects still held a great deal of their fragrance too.

Aromatic resins and gums such as frankincense and myrrh are also interesting substances. They are produced by the tree or bush by a special process known as "exudation". This is the way in which resin or gum exudes from (oozes out) of the bark itself. In the hot and dry climate where these trees and shrubs grow, one of the biggest threats to survival is water loss. Therefore, whenever there is damage to the bark or a branch drops away, the tree produces a sticky gummy mass to seal the hole. These resins and gums are also highly aromatic, and humans have been collecting them for thousands of years.

In aromatherapy wood, resin and gum essential oils are used for their protective effects on the immune and respiratory systems. They also benefit the skin; it is an interesting parallel that frankincense resin, for example, seals up "wounds" in the tree, and is also effective in healing wounds, cuts and skin-damage in humans. Making blends with these oils reconnects us through time to the ancient beginnings of aromatic use.

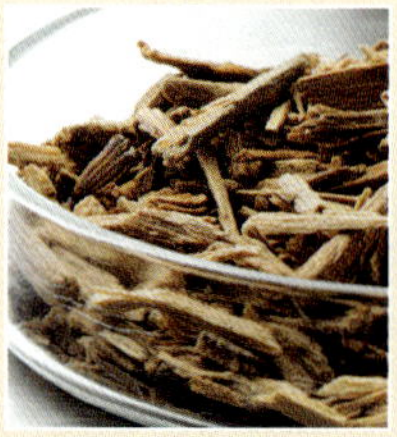

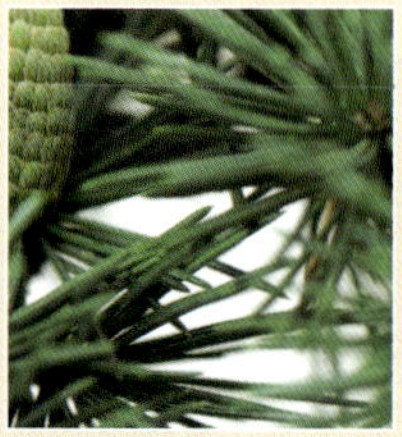

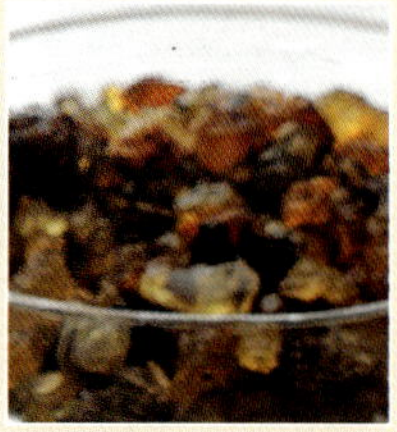

# rosewood *Aniba roseaeodora*

Rosewood essential oil has a warm woody aroma, with citrus, spicy and sweet undertones as it evaporates. A beautiful fragrance in its own right, its gentle presence creates a rounded sweetness in blends with other oils.

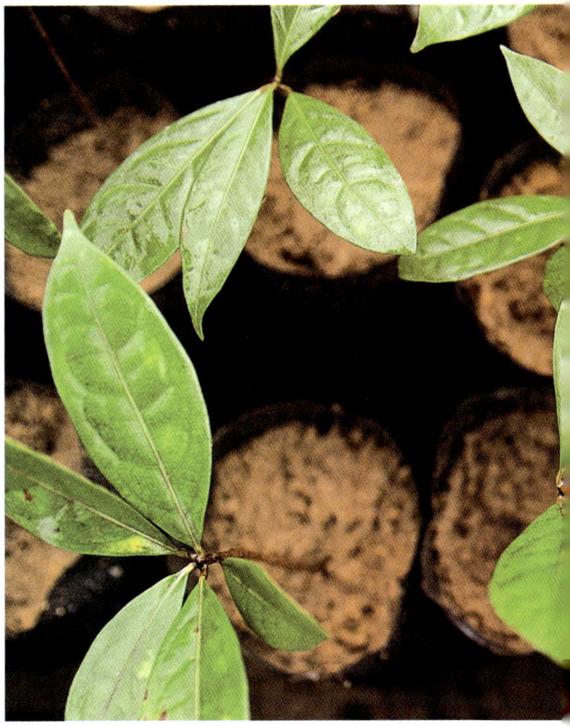

### Botanical source and background

A member of the Lauraceae plant family, which includes other aromatic trees, rosewood is a tropical evergreen native to rainforests in the Amazon basin in Brazil, Uruguay and Paraguay. It grows to about 36ft (12m) and has a reddish-coloured bark and heartwood, lance-shaped leaves, and yellow flowers. Extraction yields the greatest amount of essential oil when rosewood trees are at least 20 years old. The trees are felled extensively in Brazil, and because their timber is valuable it has been difficult to limit widespread logging. However, some rainforest areas are now protected, and Uruguay and Paraguay are making efforts to produce rosewood oil sustainably by harvesting branches and twigs rather than cutting the whole tree. In Japan rosewood is used to make chopsticks and musical instruments, and its oil is used widely in the food and perfumery industries.

### Extraction and storage

Steam distillation of the wood chippings yields a pale yellow essential oil, which will keep for up to two years in the refrigerator, and one year at cool room temperature (54°F/12°C).

### Physical and psychological effects

*Immune tonic:* can help long-term immune problems, such as chronic fatigue syndrome
*Skin-toning and rejuvenating:* soothes chapped, dry or environment-damaged skin; rejuvenates mature complexions
*Mentally-soothing:* soothes extreme nervous tension and insomnia, in children and adults
*Antidepressant:* balances pre-menstrual mood swings

### Special rosewood blends, in 4tsp (20ml) carrier oil

*Immune tonic:* Rosewood 4 drops, Mandarin 4 drops, Myrtle 2 drops
*Skin-rejuvenator:* Rosewood 2 drops, Lavender 2 drops, Rose absolute 1 drop
*Mental-soother:* Rosewood 4 drops, Roman chamomile 2 drops, Sweet orange 4 drops (use half the number of drops in 4tsp/20ml carrier for children aged 3 to 10)
*Mood-reviver:* Rosewood 4 drops, Cardamom 4 drops, Lemon 2 drops

### Safety information

Rosewood essential oil is non-toxic, non-irritating and non-sensitizing.

# frankincense *Boswellia carterii*

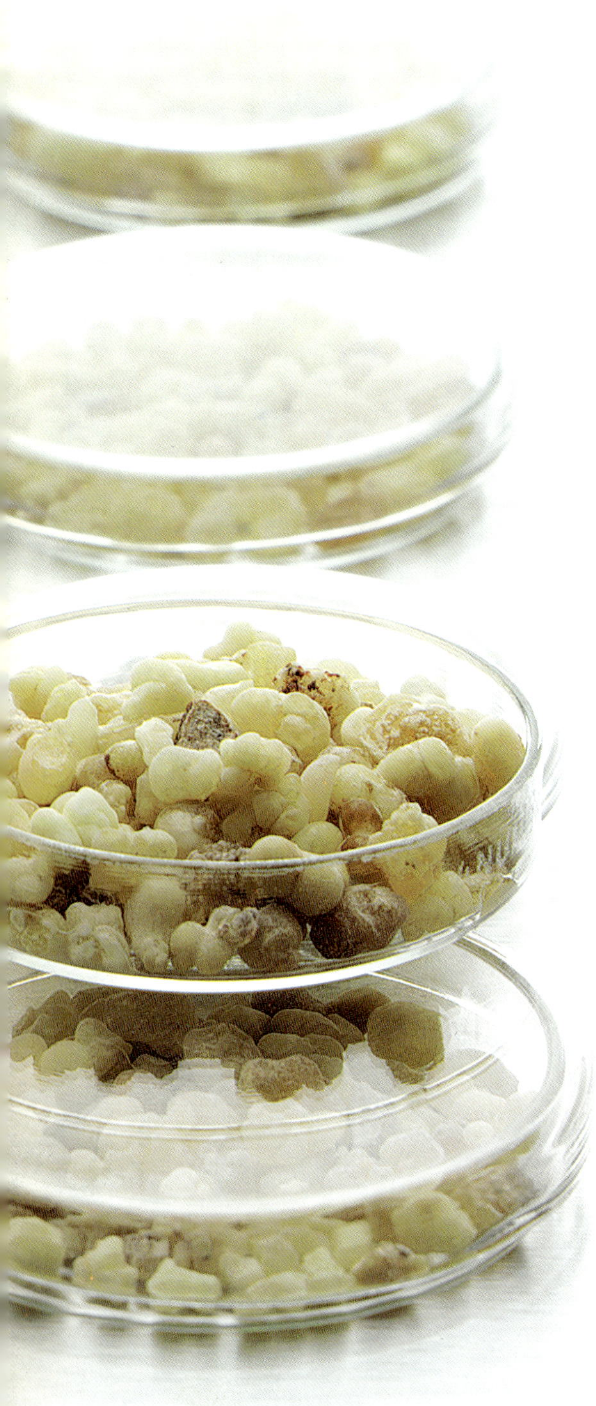

Frankincense essential oil has an uplifting, sharp and fresh aroma, becoming richer, warmer and sweeter as it evaporates. It is a fragrance that helps to create a meditative state of peace and calm.

### Botanical source and background

Frankincense belongs to the Burseraceae family and is found in Africa and the Middle East. The tree can grow up to 30ft (10m) tall and thrives in rocky, dry areas of desert or mountains. Making deliberate incisions into the bark causes its milky-white or yellowish resin to ooze out. This hardens into drop-like shapes called "tears", which are ground up for use as incense or for distillation of the essential oil. Frankincense has been used since ancient times in India, China, Egypt, the Middle East and Europe in medicine, cosmetics, embalming and ritual. The name comes from the old French *franc encens*, meaning "true incense". Frankincense was one of the gifts brought to the infant Christ by the Three Wise Men; its symbolic meaning was a recognition of the spiritual inheritance of the Holy Child. It is still burned as incense in the Roman Catholic and Orthodox churches today.

### Extraction and storage

Steam distillation of the ground resin yields a pale yellow essential oil, which will last up to two years in the refrigerator, and one year at cool room temperature (54°F/12°C).

### Physical and psychological effects

*Skin-rejuvenator:* restores dry, tired, environment-damaged or mature skin, and improves the appearance of fine lines
*Respiratory tonic*: calms and slows down the breath, clears mucus and soothes coughs
*Immune-boosting:* improves resistance to bacterial or viral infections
*Uplifting:* inspires the mind

### Special frankincense blends, in 4tsp (20ml) carrier oil

*Facial skin-rejuvenator:* Frankincense 2 drops, Rosewood 2 drops, Rose absolute 1 drop
*Special mature facial treat:* Frankincense 2 drops, Rose otto 1 drop, Neroli 1 drop, Sandalwood 1 drop
*Immune tonic:* Frankincense 4 drops, Lemon 4 drops, Ginger 2 drops
*Spiritual inspiration:* Frankincense 4 drops, Grapefruit 4 drops, Myrtle 2 drops

### Safety information

Frankincense esssential oil is non-toxic, non-irritating and non-sensitizing.

# atlas cedarwood *Cedrus atlantica*

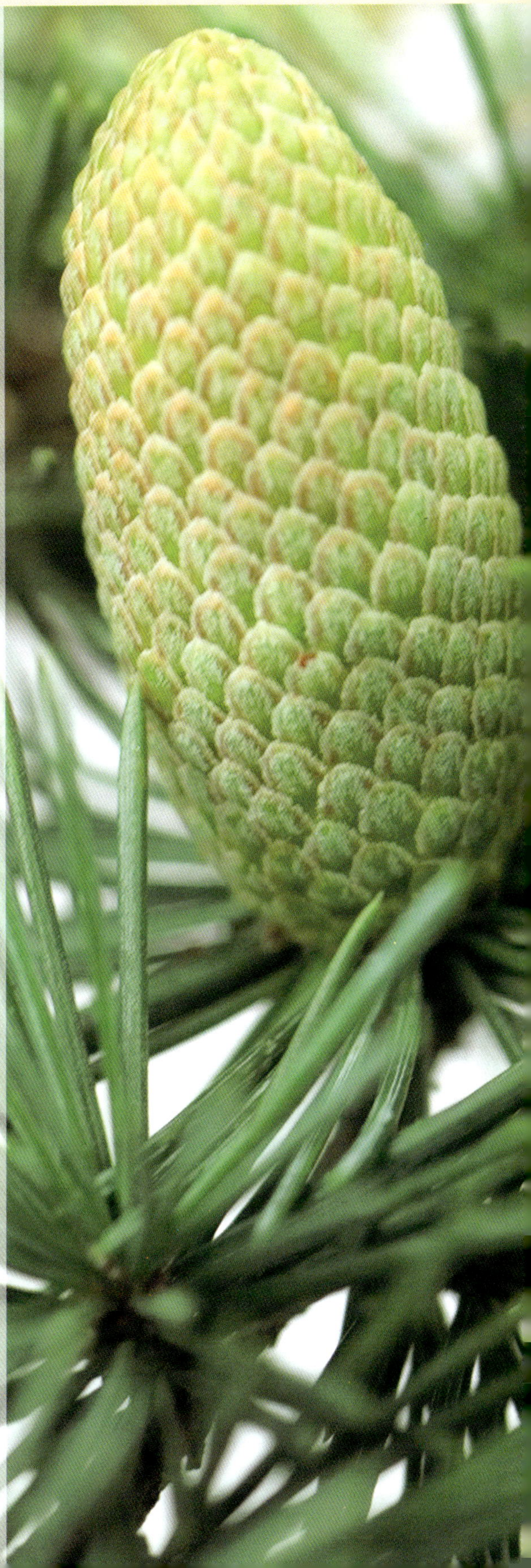

Atlas cedarwood has a beautiful resiny, sweet aroma, with deeper woody undertones. It becomes much richer and softer on evaporation, encouraging a calm mind and a sense of tranquillity.

### Botanical source and background

A member of the extensive Pinaceae family of evergreen trees, Atlas cedarwood is native to the Atlas mountains of Morocco, North Africa. It grows to a maximum height of 120ft (40m), and has sweeping branches with greyish-green needles and oval cones, dripping with fragrant resin. Atlas cedarwood essential oil is found in the red heartwood of the branches and the trunk. The Ancient Egyptians used the resin extensively as an incense, a cosmetic and in the embalming process. It was also favoured by the Ancient Greeks to help preserve bodies – they associated it with immortality. Today, the perfume industry uses it in the formulation of mens' fragrances.

### Extraction and storage

Steam distillation of the wood yields a golden yellow essential oil, which will keep for up to two years in the refrigerator, and up to one year at cool room temperature (54°F/12°C).

### Physical and psychological effects

*Skin-rejuvenator:* brightens tired and dull complexions
*Respiratory tonic:* soothes and eases coughs, bronchitis, catarrh and asthma
*Circulatory tonic:* improves circulation, eases aches and pains
*Nervous restorative:* supports overstrained nerves

### Special Atlas cedarwood blends, in 4tsp (20ml) carrier oil

*Luxury facial-reviver:* Atlas cedarwood 2 drops, Myrrh 1 drop, Rose otto 1 drop, Frankincense 1 drop
*Respiratory-soother:* Atlas cedarwood 4 drops, Myrtle 4 drops, Cypress 2 drops
*Circulatory tonic:* Atlas cedarwood 4 drops, May chang 4 drops, Ginger 4 drops
*Mental-support:* Atlas cedarwood 4 drops, Mandarin 4 drops, Rosewood 2 drops

### Safety information

Atlas cedarwood is non-toxic, non-irritating and non-sensitizing. However, be aware that essential oils sold in the US as Texan or Virginian cedarwood are different botanical species to Atlas cedarwood and are not recommended.

# myrrh *Commiphora myrrha*

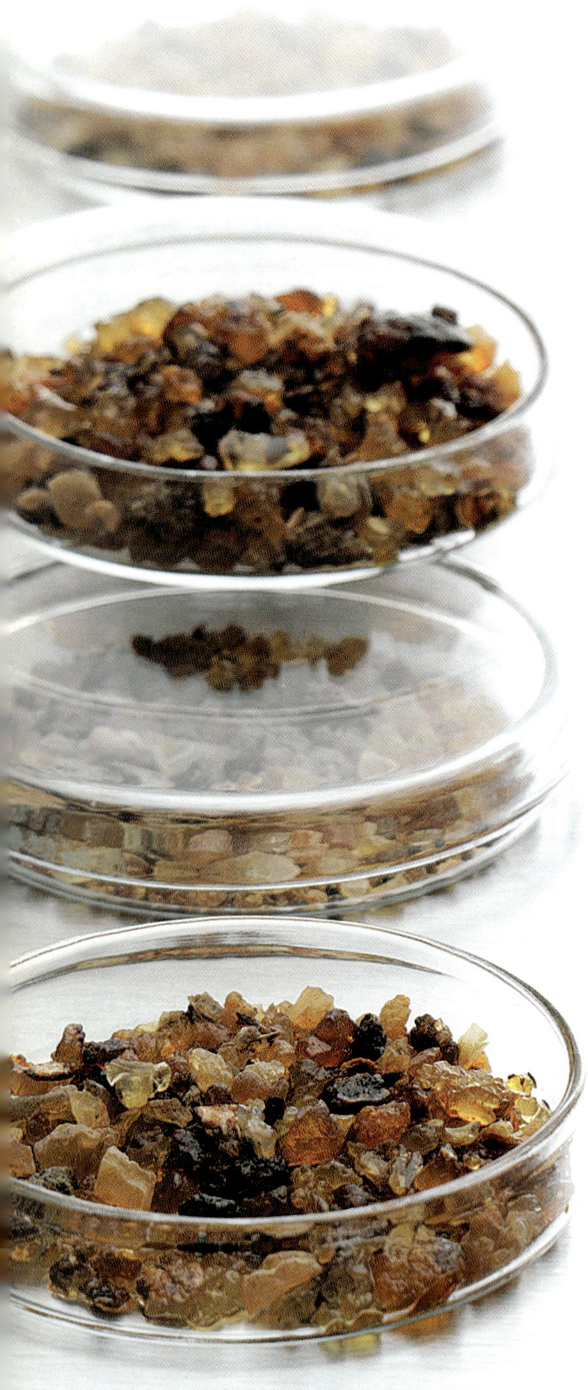

Myrrh has a highly unusual fragrance – sharp and medicinal to begin, then becoming richer, sweeter and intriguingly smoky as it evaporates. It was regarded as one of the finest perfumes in Ancient Egypt.

## Botanical source and background

A member of the Burseraceae plant family, the Myrrh bush grows mainly in Somalia, Yemen and Saudi Arabia. Around 9ft (3m) tall, it has long sharp thorns, small three-lobed leaves and white flowers. Cuts made into its bark encourage the bush to produce thick yellow gum, which dries to an orange-brown colour and is collected for making incense and oil. Myrrh is an ancient fragrance ingredient, used in cosmetics, embalming, perfumery and religious rites for 4,000 years. It was one of the gifts of the Wise Men at the birth of Christ, and symbolized the sacred oils which anoint a king; it was also used to embalm him at his death. Its name is said to derive from the Arabic *mur*, meaning "bitter", which describes the smell and the taste of the gum. Western European herbal tradition has valued myrrh for centuries as an antiseptic protection against infectious diseases.

## Extraction and storage

Steam distillation of myrrh gum yields a pale yellow essential oil, which will last up to two years in the refrigerator, and one year at cool room temperature (54°F/12°C). As the oil degrades it becomes much thicker.

## Physical and psychological effects

*Respiratory tonic:* helps chesty coughs or bronchitis
*Skin-healer:* regenerates deeply cracked, wounded or damaged skin
*Menstrual tonic:* eases period pain
*Mentally calming:* soothes and steadies the mind, easing anxiety and tension

## Special myrrh blends, in 4tsp (20ml) carrier oil

*Respiratory tonic:* Myrrh 4 drops, Atlas cedarwood 4 drops, Spanish sage 2 drops
*Damaged-skin repair:* Myrrh 4 drops, German chamomile 4 drops, Frankincense 2 drops
*Menstrual-soother:* Myrrh 4 drops, Sweet marjoram 4 drops, Vetiver 2 drops
*Emotional-soother:* Myrrh 2 drops, Sweet orange 4 drops, Sandalwood 4 drops

## Safety information

Myrrh is non-toxic, non-irritant and non-sensitizing. As it is a strong tonic to the uterus, its use is not recommended during pregnancy.

# sandalwood *Santalum album*

Sandalwood oil has a sweet, light woody aroma, becoming richer and warmer as it evaporates. Its soft spicy notes leave a lingering fragrance on the skin, which is exotic and seductive.

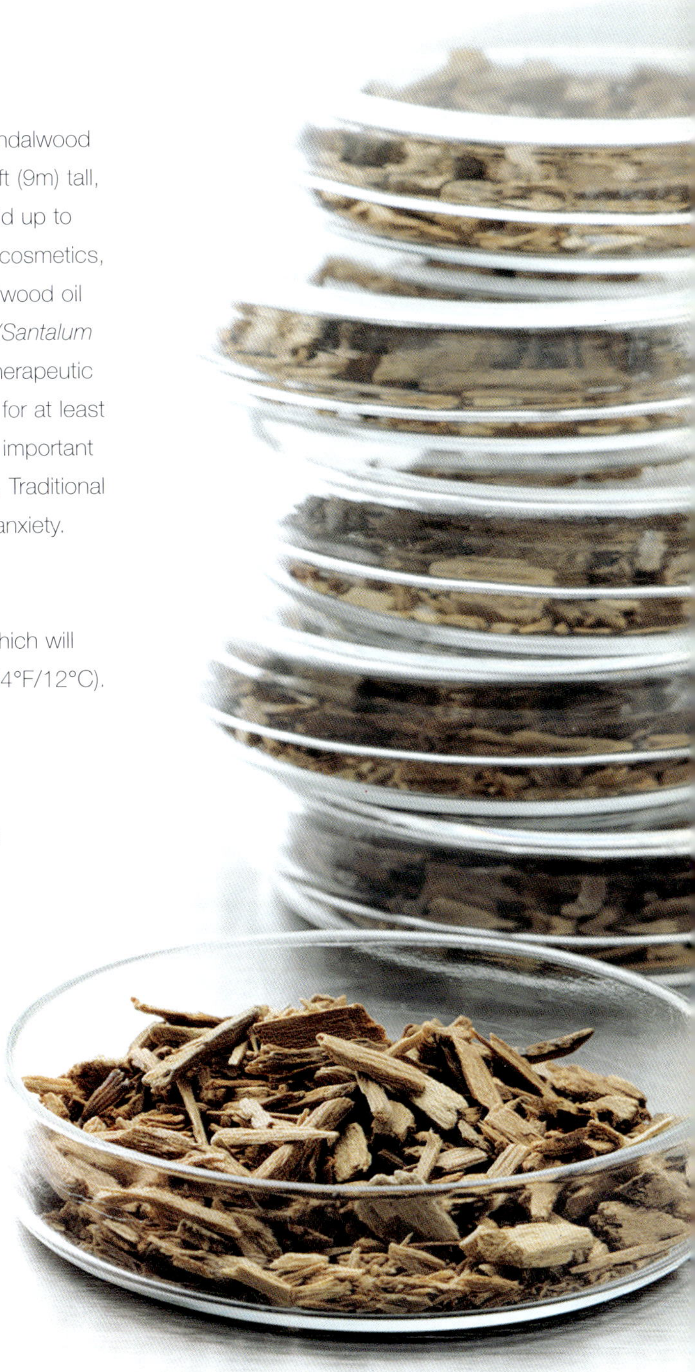

### Botanical source and background

The sandalwood tree belongs to the Santalaceae family, and the best-quality sandalwood oil comes from the Mysore region of India near Bangalore. A small tree up to 27ft (9m) tall, the sandalwood must mature for at least 30 years to allow its essential oil to build up to full intensity. Once felled, the tree's aromatic timber is used in furniture, incense, cosmetics, perfumery and essential-oil production. A world shortage of quality Indian sandalwood oil has led producers to investigate other species, such as Australian sandalwood *(Santalum spicatum)*, but these do not have the rich odour of the Indian oil nor the same therapeutic effects. Indian sandalwood is an ancient perfumery material that has been used for at least 4,000 years. It remains a key element in Hindu religious practice, used to scent important ceremonies. In Ancient Egypt sandalwood was used in incense and embalming. Traditional Tibetan and Chinese Medicine uses sandalwood to purify the body and relieve anxiety.

### Extraction and storage

Steam distillation of sandalwood chips yields a thick, pale yellow essential oil, which will last up to two years in the refrigerator, and one year at cool room temperature (54°F/12°C).

### Physical and psychological effects

*Skin-toning:* tones and smoothes dry, mature or environment-damaged skin
*Respiratory tonic:* helps all throat and respiratory infections, coughs and asthma
*Immune-boosting:* improves resistance to infections
*Detoxifying:* improves lymphatic flow, helping the removal of toxins
*Mentally-calming:* is soothing, gentle and enveloping to the mind

### Special sandalwood blends, in 4tsp (20ml) carrier oil

*Super-facial tonic:* Sandalwood 2 drops, Neroli 1 drop, Frankincense 2 drops
*Immune tonic:* Sandalwood 4 drops, Cardamom 4 drops, Lemon 2 drops
*Detoxifier:* Sandalwood 4 drops, Fennel 4 drops, Grapefruit 2 drops
*Mental-soother:* Sandalwood 4 drops, Atlas cedarwood 4 drops, Myrtle 2 drops

### Safety information

Sandalwood essential oil is non-toxic, non-irritating and non-sensitizing.

# leaf and root oils

Around half of the essential oils in an aromatherapist's kit usually come from leaves, the commonest source of aromatic plant tissue. These have cleansing properties. Root oils are valuable too, and are used for their warming and strengthening effects.

Anthropologists speculate that our early ancestors roamed the Earth for thousands of years, foraging as they went, tasting, testing and learning how to use countless leaves as bandages, medicines, flavourings and ritual garlands. Guided by keen noses, these hunter-gatherers must have been particularly attracted to aromatic plants. In more recent times, research among ethnic peoples who still live close to the land has shown how much they continue to use aromatic leaves. The leaves are variously chewed, drunk as teas, rubbed onto the body as perfume or insect repellent, soaked and pounded into pastes for wound-healing, or draped around the neck in important ceremonies.

In any plant the leaves are responsible for photosynthesis – the vital process that generates food and energy for the plant. Photosynthesis involves a reaction between sunlight and certain cells in the leaf, known as chloroplasts, which have evolved a unique way of turning that light into sugars, the building blocks for plant tissue. Some plant species, for reasons that are still unclear, have also evolved special types of cells either within their leaf structure, or slightly outside it in microscopic velvety hairs; these cells are where essential oils build up until the leaf gives off a powerful aroma. Overall, only relatively few plant families on the planet are actually aromatic – no more than 1 to 2 per cent of the total number of known groups – which begs the question, why have these particular plants evolved as producers of essential oils, and not others? There is no definite answer; opinions from botanists seem to be that the oils might be waste products, or that they may well make the plant more attractive to birds and animals and thereby aid pollination, or that they may repel certain insects.

Many leaf essential oils used in aromatherapy come from the family group Labiatae. These are plants traditionally of Mediterranean origin such as rosemary, peppermint, basil or thyme. They grow best in extreme heat and sunlight and are more aromatic the hotter the climate. Leaf oils often have wonderful fresh pungent aromas which help respiratory and immune problems. Given that leaves also help a plant to "breathe" – to exchange oxygen and carbon dioxide by another important plant process called transpiration – this is an interesting parallel. In aromatherapy we also value the leaf oils for their fresh, cleansing properties.

Root essential oils are found in plant tissues which grow underground. They often occur in exotic plant species such as ginger, turmeric or vetiver. These plants come from tropical climates where the insects and grubs in the soil can be extremely voracious. Essential oils in the roots may well protect these plants from insect attack, helping them to survive. Root oils are used in aromatherapy for warming and strengthening the body; they tend to have earthy or richly spicy aromas.

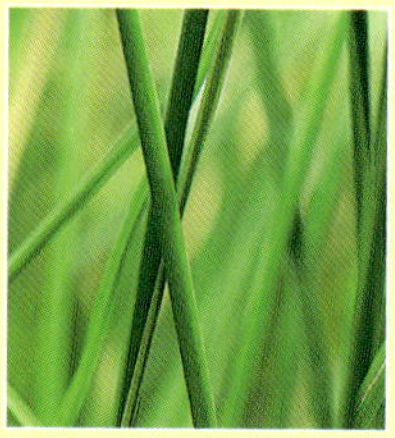

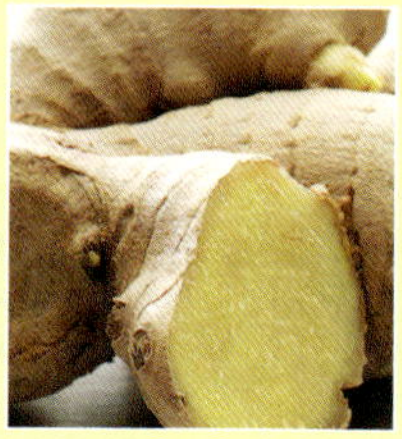

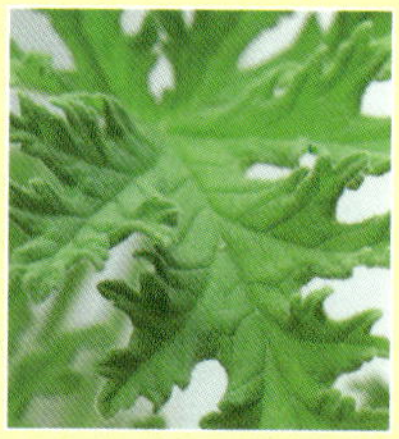

# yarrow *Achillea millefolium*

Yarrow essential oil has a creamy-sweet, cool, slightly sharp aroma with herbaceous and mildly camphoraceous undertones, growing sweeter again as it evaporates.

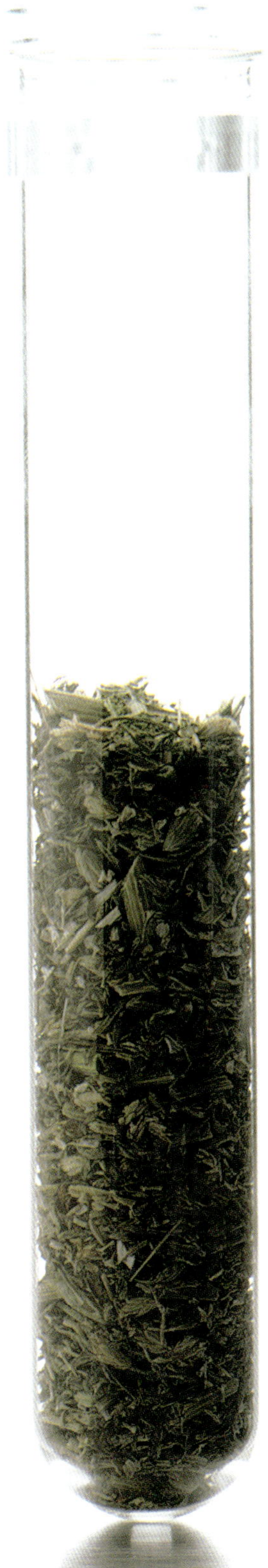

### Botanical source and background

Yarrow belongs to the large Compositae family, whose flowers all have a daisy-like appearance. It grows wild across a vast area that includes the UK, mainland Europe and Asia; and has been introduced into North America, Australia and New Zealand. Yarrow oil is produced in Germany and Hungary. A perennial herb growing up to 2ft (60cm) tall, yarrow has dark green, feathery leaves and flat heads of tiny white flowers. Its botanical name *Achillea* is linked to the Ancient Greek hero Achilles, who was said to have used the herb to stop wounds from bleeding. In ancient times, other names for the plant were "soldiers' woundwort" or "bloodwort". In the 17th century, English herbalist Nicholas Culpeper used yarrow tea to improve sleep. Today, herbalists still recommended a blended tea made from dried yarrow, peppermint and elderflower as an effective remedy for flu.

### Extraction and storage

Steam distillation of dried yarrow yields a dark blue essential oil, which is rich in an anti-inflammatory constituent called azulene. Yarrow oil will last up to two years in the refrigerator, and up to one year at cool room temperature (54°F/12°C).

### Physical and psychological effects

*Anti-inflammatory:* reduces inflammation, calms and repairs sore or reddened skin
*Digestive tonic:* soothes stomach aches, digestive cramps and indigestion
*Anti-allergic:* calms skin reactions such as nettle rash, heat rash and allergies
*Wound-healing:* heals deeply cracked or damaged skin
*Emotionally-soothing:* calms angry, inflamed emotions

### Special yarrow blends, in 4tsp (20ml) carrier oil

*Skin-soother:* Yarrow 2 drops, Roman chamomile 4 drops, Lavender 4 drops
*Digestive-soother:* Yarrow 2 drops, Turmeric 4 drops, May chang 4 drops
*Anti-itch:* Yarrow 2 drops, Rose otto 2 drops
*Damaged-skin repair:* Yarrow 2 drops, Myrrh 4 drops, Frankincense 4 drops

### Safety information

Do not use on sufferers of epilepsy. Otherwise non-toxic, non-irritating and non-sensitizing.

# angelica *Angelica archangelica*

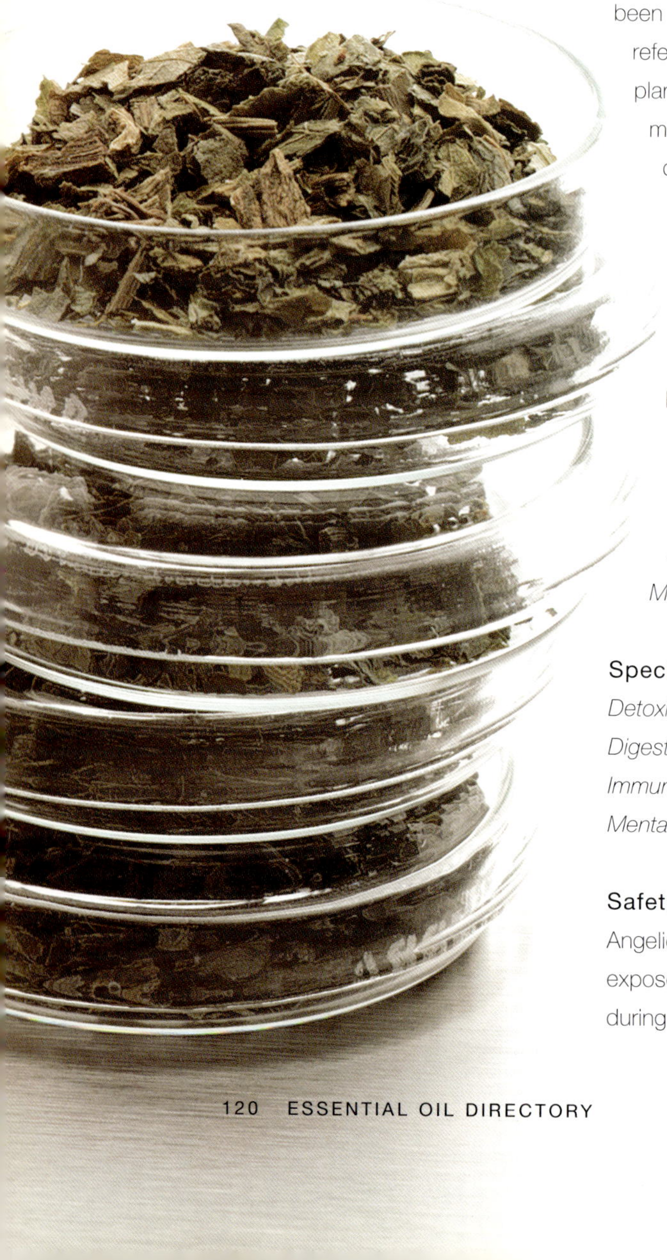

Angelica essential oil has a warm, delicate and sweet aroma with hints of aniseed and spice, slightly woody and sweet as it evaporates. Subtle and light, it is gentle and soothing to the spirit.

### Botanical source and background

A member of the Umbelliferae plant family, angelica is found in Germany, France, Holland and Eastern Europe, both as a cultivated plant and growing wild in moist ditches or on riverbanks. It is a majestic aromatic plant up to 6ft (2m) tall, with thick ridged stems, toothed dark green leaves and dramatic globular flower heads, producing whitish blooms in early summer. The essential oil is taken from the dried roots. In the West, angelica has been used for centuries to purify the blood and fight infection. Its Latin name *archangelica* refers to the Archangel Michael, whose feast day of May 8 usually coincides with the plant flowering. Angelica stems were also candied by boiling in sugar to eat as a sweet-meat. Western European herbal medicine values the roots as a stomach tonic and diuretic remedy.

### Extraction and storage

Steam distillation of the dried roots yields a colourless essential oil, which will last up to two years in the refrigerator, or one year at cool room temperature (54°F/12°C).

### Physical and psychological effects

*Detoxifying:* eases rheumatism or gout; helps to improve the appearance of cellulite.
*Digestive tonic:* is beneficial for indigestion, constipation, stomach aches and irregular bowel rhythm
*Immune-boosting:* builds resistance to bacterial and viral infections
*Mentally-uplifting:* uplifts negative emotions; eases nervous tension

### Special angelica blends, in 4tsp (20ml) carrier oil

*Detoxifier:* Angelica 2 drops, Fennel 4 drops, Grapefruit 4 drops
*Digestive tonic:* Angelica 2 drops, Mandarin 4 drops, Coriander seed 4 drops
*Immune tonic:* Angelica 2 drops, Manuka 4 drops, Lemon 4 drops
*Mental-rejuvenator:* Angelica 2 drops, Myrtle 4 drops, Sweet orange 4 drops

### Safety information

Angelica is phototoxic; if you massage a blend containing angelica onto the skin, do not expose the skin to UV light for 12 hours following application. The oil is best avoided during pregnancy because it can stimulate the uterus.

# petitgrain *Citrus aurantium*

Petitgrain, also known as orange leaf, produces essential oil with a fresh, green and citrusy aroma, with sweet and slightly warm undertones, woodier and more herbaceous as it evaporates. It is light and refreshing.

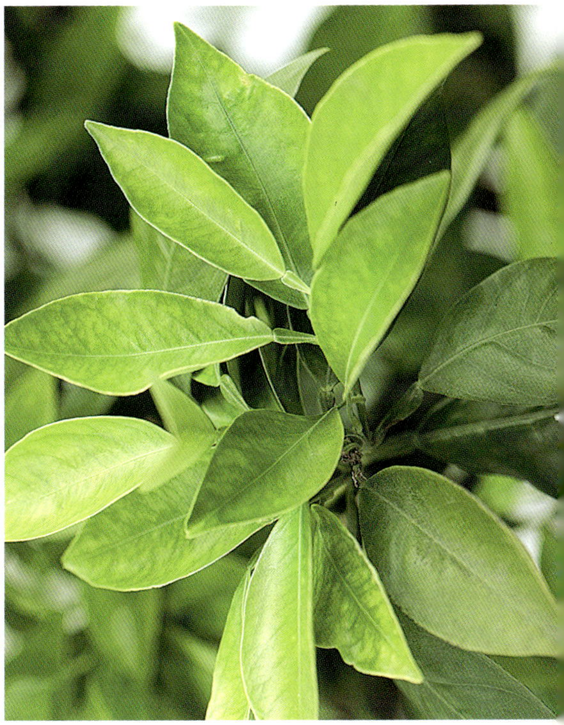

### Botanical source and background

Petitgrain comes from the bitter orange tree which is a member of the Rutaceae family. The oil is produced in France and Paraguay. The bitter orange is an attractive evergreen growing up to 30ft (10m) tall, with glossy, dark green, aromatic leaves, fragrant creamy white flowers (which are the source of neroli essential oil) and wrinkled greenish-orange fruit. The French *petitgrain* means "little grain"; this may refer to the visible essential oil sacs in the leaves of the tree which show up as little spots when held up to the light. The bitter orange tree is originally from China; it was introduced into Europe and cultivated by early Arab traders. Petitgrain has been used as a fragrance ingredient since the 18th century. It is one of the main notes in the original eau-de-Cologne formula, along with lavender, bergamot, orange, rosemary and neroli. Petitgrain is used extensively to scent soaps, bath products, cosmetics and perfumes. It is pleasing to both men and women.

### Extraction and storage

Steam distillation of the leaves yields a very pale yellow essential oil. It will last up to two years in the refrigerator, and up to one year at cool room temperature (54°F/12°C).

### Physical and psychological effects

*Oily-skin tonic:* tones oily and combination skins
*Skin antiseptic:* heals acne or blemished skin; dries up spots and helps prevent scarring
*Digestive tonic:* eases indigestion, wind, constipation, and stomach aches that have been made worse by emotional stress
*Nervous restorative:* calms the nerves and helps relieve insomnia

### Special petitgrain blends, in 4tsp (20ml) carrier oil

*Oily-skin treatment:* Petitgrain 2 drops, Geranium 2 drops, Mandarin 1 drop
*Skin-blemish treatment:* Petitgrain 2 drops, Tea tree 2 drops, Myrrh 1 drop
*Digestive-soother:* Petitgrain 4 drops, Fennel 2 drops, Grapefruit 4 drops
*Mental-soother:* Petitgrain 4 drops, Neroli 2 drops, Lavender 4 drops

### Safety information

Petitgrain essential oil is non-toxic, non-irritating and non-sensitizing.

# cypress *Cupressus sempervirens*

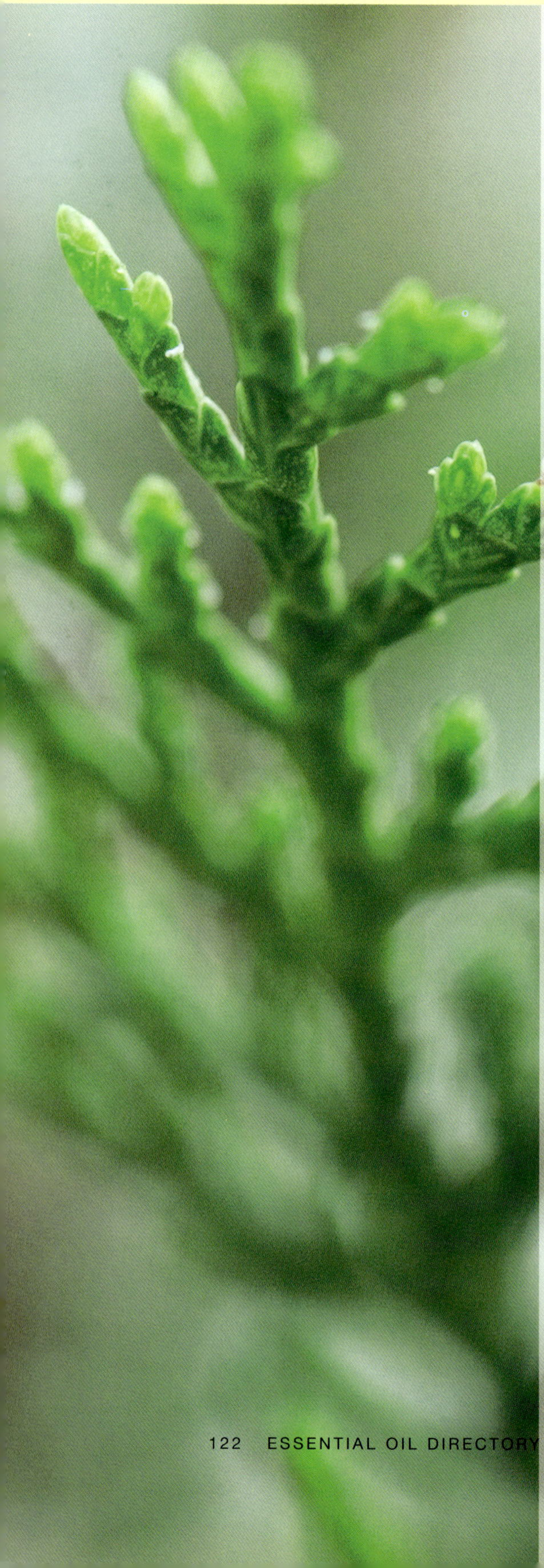

Cypress essential oil has a warm woody aroma, and is sweet and slightly smoky, with earthy and gently spicy undertones. It is a long-lasting fragrance, adding deep and evocative notes to aromatic combinations.

### Botanical source and background

A member of the ancient Cupressaceae family of evergreen trees and shrubs, cypress is native to the eastern Mediterranean region, and its essential oil is produced in Spain, Morocco and France. Today, it grows all over Europe and as far east as Tibet and China. The trees are highly aromatic and conical-shaped. The cypresses are one of the oldest known plant families; remains of ancestral varieties have been found in rocks dating back four million years. Some cypresses standing today are more than 2,000 years old. This longevity led them to be considered as gateways to the underworld in old Mediterranean folklore. Cypress branches have traditionally been burned as incense, and the leaves and cones were used in Ancient Greece to treat wounds, hemorrhoids and internal bleeding. In Western herbal tradition, cypress is used to help kidney problems and excess menstrual bleeding. It is also a cleansing and purifying ingredient in Traditional Chinese Medicine.

### Extraction and storage

Steam distillation of the leaves and twigs yields a yellow essential oil. It will keep up to one year in the refrigerator, and up to six months at cool room temperature (54°F/12°C); old cypress oil becomes thick and viscous.

### Physical and psychological effects

*Diuretic:* clears excess fluid and improves the appearance of cellulite
*Menstrual tonic:* tones the uterus and helps reduce excess menstrual bleeding
*Expectorant:* helps tight and sore coughs
*Mentally-soothing:* calms excess mental stress and nervous tension

### Special cypress blends, in 4tsp (20ml) carrier oil

*Detoxifier:* Cypress 4 drops, Fennel 2 drops, Grapefruit 4 drops
*Menstrual-balancer:* Cypress 4 drops, Clary sage 2 drops, Sweet orange 4 drops
*Cough-comforter:* Cypress 4 drops, Cardamom 4 drops, Ginger 2 drops
*Mental-soother:* Cypress 4 drops, Lavender 4 drops, Mandarin 2 drops

### Safety information

Cypress essential oil is non-toxic, non-irritating and non-sensitizing.

# turmeric *Curcuma longa*

Turmeric essential oil is soft, warm and gently spicy with a more earthy and subtle undertone, and becomes sweeter on evaporation. It is immediately reminiscent of moist tropical vegetation.

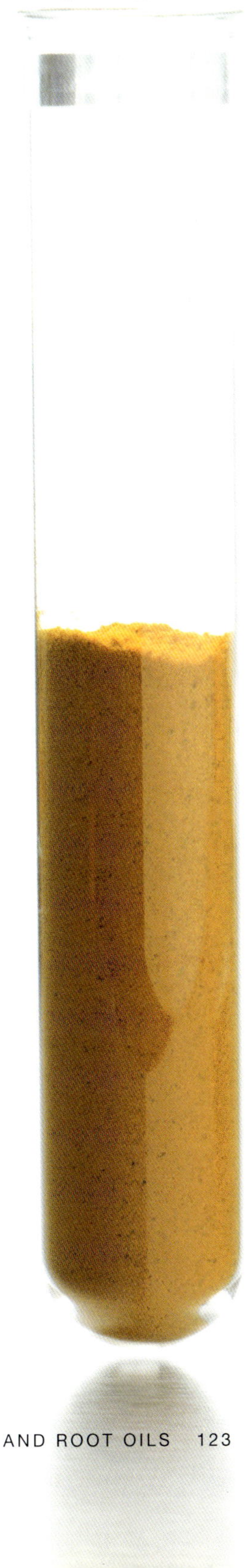

### Botanical source and background

Turmeric belongs to the Zingiberaceae family, which includes ginger. Native to southern Asia, its essential oil is distilled in China, India and Japan. Turmeric has long elegant green stalks up to 3ft (1m) tall, with large, rich green, lance-shaped leaves. The essential oil is found in the fleshy root, which is bright yellow-orange in colour when freshly cut open. Turmeric root is rich in vitamins and minerals as well as aromatic compounds. Dried ground turmeric root has been used as a spice and medicine in the East for thousands of years. In Chinese medicine it is traditionally used to treat stomach disorders, bruising and open sores on the skin. Indian Ayurvedic tradition uses turmeric as an internal cleanser, especially for toning the kidneys, and as a popular cooking ingredient which helps to stimulate healthy digestion. Current research in India suggests that including turmeric in the diet may help to prevent serious bowel disorders. Turmeric root is also used as a strong yellow dye in Far Eastern countries.

### Extraction and storage

The root is dried before distillation; the essential oil is bright yellow. It will last up to two years in the refrigerator, or up to one year at cool room temperature (54°F/12°C).

### Physical and psychological effects

*Digestive tonic:* eases indigestion, stomach cramps, constipation and sluggish digestion
*Diuretic:* stimulates the body to detoxify itself
*Damaged-skin healer:* speeds up repair of damaged skin or ulcers
*Immune-boosting:* builds resistance to immune infections

### Special turmeric blends, in 4tsp (20ml) carrier oil

*Digestive tonic:* Turmeric 2 drops, Coriander seed 4 drops, Sweet orange 4 drops
*Anti-cellulite:* Turmeric 4 drops, Grapefruit 4 drops, Juniper berry 2 drops
*Skin repair:* Turmeric 2 drops, German chamomile 2 drops, Frankincense 6 drops
*Immune tonic:* Turmeric 4 drops, Black pepper 2 drops, Mandarin 4 drops

### Safety information

Turmeric oil is non-toxic, non-irritating and non-sensitizing.

# lemongrass *Cymbopogon citratus*

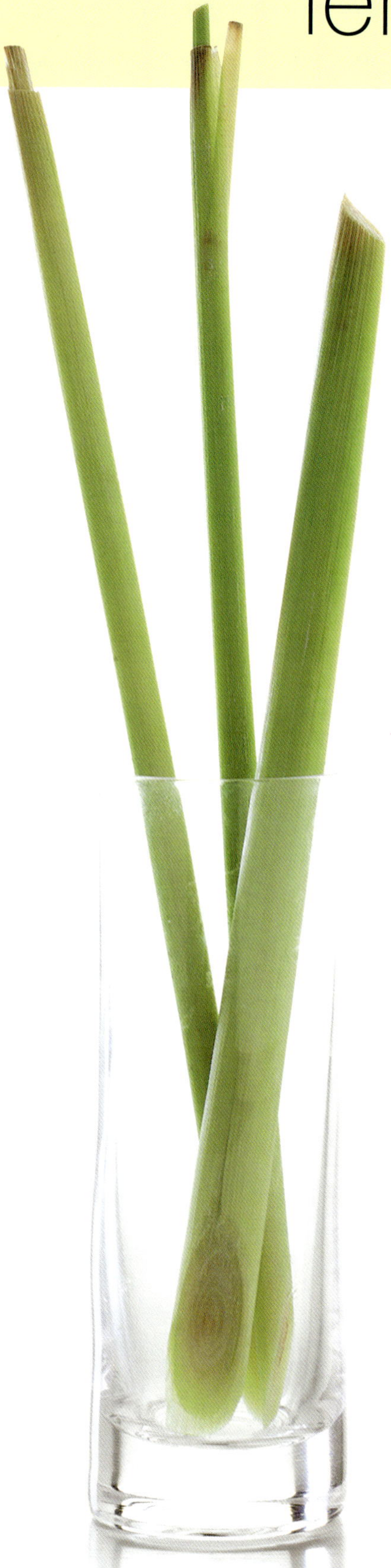

Lemongrass essential oil has a sweet, sherbet-like and zesty aroma, with powerful lemony and oily undertones. It has a long-lasting fragrance that is fresh, mouth-watering, citrusy and light.

## Botanical source and background

A member of the Gramineae family of grasses, this type of lemongrass is known as "West Indian Lemongrass". It is grown commercially in Madagascar, Brazil, Malaysia and Vietnam and is used to produce the most commonly available lemongrass essential oil. Another variety, *Cymbopogon flexuosus* from India, is also used in aromatherapy and has similar effects. A scented tropical grass up to 5ft (1.5m) tall, West Indian lemongrass has aromatic lemon-scented blades which produce essential oil. Young shoots are a medical remedy and a flavouring in many eastern countries such as China and Malaysia. In Thai cooking, lemongrass is finely chopped and added to many recipes. Traditional Chinese Medicine uses lemongrass to treat headaches, colds, stomach pains and rheumatism. Today, the oil is used as a fragrance ingredient in many foods, drinks and personal-care products. In India, lemongrass is a remedy for fevers and other infectious diseases, and an insect repellent.

## Extraction and storage

Steam distillation of the grass yields a pale yellow essential oil, which will last up to two years in the refrigerator, and up to one year at cool room temperature (54°F/12°C).

## Physical and psychological effects

*Analgesic:* helps stiffness, muscular aches and pains, strains and muscle spasm
*Digestive tonic:* eases constipation and indigestion
*Insect repellent:* can be used preventively against mosquito bites
*Nervous restorative:* refreshes and revives the nerves; eases mental stress

## Special lemongrass blends, in 4tsp (20ml) carrier oil

*Muscle treatment:* Lemongrass 2 drops, Myrtle 4 drops, Cardamom 4 drops
*Digestive-soother:* Lemongrass 2 drops, Coriander seed 4 drops, Turmeric 4 drops
*Insect repellent:* Lemongrass 2 drops, Patchouli 2 drops, Lavender 6 drops
*Mental-reviver:* Lemongrass 2 drops, Basil 4 drops, Myrtle 4 drops

## Safety information

Lemongrass should not be used on sensitive, damaged or allergy-prone skin, nor on children under 10. It is a strong oil so never exceed the stated number of drops in blends.

# palmarosa *Cymbopogon martinii*

Palmarosa essential oil has an intensely sweet and rosy aroma with a light, green freshness as it evaporates. It has a subtle and gentle quality, soothing and soft, and blends well with many other fragrances.

### Botanical source and background

Belonging to the Gramineae family of grasses, palmarosa is native to India, where it grows wild and is also known as "rosha". It has been introduced for cultivation to Africa, Brazil and Indonesia where it is now produced commercially. Palmarosa is a scented tropical grass with slender stems and blades and a sweet and rosy aroma. In traditional Indian medicine, the leaves are used as a treatment for rheumatism and other nerve pains. The oil found its way to Europe via the trade routes between India and ancient Persia; it became known as "Indian geranium oil" because of its sweet rosy fragrance. In India it is used to make sweet incense blends. Palmarosa oil is used today in cosmetic and perfumery formulations and as a sweet fragrance in soap.

### Extraction and storage

Steam distillation of the grass produces a very pale essential oil, which will keep up to two years in the refrigerator, and one year at cool room temperature (54°F/12°C).

### Physical and psychological effects

*Skin-hydrating:* restores moisture in excessively dry or delicate skins
*Skin-rejuvenating:* restores suppleness and elasticity to tired or mature complexions
*Skin-clearing:* is gently antiseptic on skin infections such as acne, helping spots to heal with minimum scarring
*Mentally-soothing:* calms severe emotional tension or stress

### Special palmarosa blends, in 4tsp (20ml) carrier oil

*Luxury skin moisturiser:* Palmarosa 2 drops, Neroli 2 drops, Carrot seed 1 drop
*Mature skin tonic:* Palmarosa 2 drops, Patchouli 1 drop, Jasmine 2 drops
*Special facial-blemish treatment:* Palmarosa 2 drops, Myrrh 1 drop, Frankincense 2 drops
*Immune tonic:* Palmarosa 4 drops, Lemon 4 drops, Manuka 2 drops
*Mental-soother:* Palmarosa 4 drops, Sweet orange 4 drops, Roman chamomile 2 drops

### Safety information

Palmarosa essential oil is non-toxic, non-irritating and non-sensitizing.

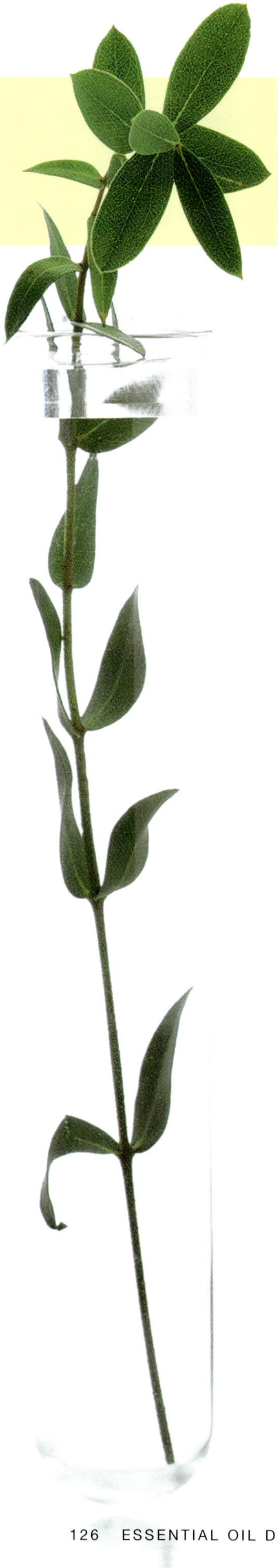

# eucalyptus *Eucalyptus globulus*

Eucalyptus essential oil has a sharp, medicinal and green aroma with penetrating, fresh camphoraceous notes, then woodier undertones as it evaporates. Its bracing fragrance instantly clears the head and chest.

## Botanical source and background

A member of the Myrtaceae family, which includes many aromatic trees, eucalyptus originated in Australia, where there are more than 500 known species, and has been introduced to Spain, Portugal and China. It is a tall evergreen tree with greenish-grey leaves, and can grow up to 200ft (65m) in good conditions. *Eucalyptus globulus* is the variety that provides the vast majority of eucalyptus essential oil used worldwide. Eucalyptus is a valuable traditional remedy in Australia. Soaking the leaves in boiling water gives off a vapour which helps coughs and chest congestion. This infusion is also used as an antiseptic wash for cuts, wounds and insect bites, and is reputed to help the symptoms of malaria. The eucalyptus oil industry in Australia began in the late 19th century, and the antiviral and antiseptic effects of the oil were much in demand during the First World War.

## Extraction and storage

Steam distillation of the leaves and young twigs yields a colourless essential oil. It lasts for up to two years in the refrigerator, and one year at cool room temperature (54°F/12°C).

## Physical and psychological effects

*Circulatory stimulant:* warms cold hands and feet or chilly limbs
*Analgesic:* eases backache, muscle spasms and pulls, and sports-related injuries
*Expectorant:* eases coughs, chest congestion and tightness
*Wound-healing:* heals damaged skin, cuts and grazes and minor wounds
*Mentally-stimulating:* invigorates the mind and improves concentration

## Special eucalyptus blends, in 4tsp (20ml) carrier oil

*Muscle-ache treatment:* Eucalyptus 2 drops, Black pepper 4 drops, May chang 4 drops
*Chest relief:* Eucalyptus 2 drops, Atlas cedarwood 4 drops, Lemon 4 drops
*Wound-healer:* Eucalyptus 2 drops, Tea tree 4 drops, Myrrh 4 drops
*Mental-rejuvenator:* Eucalyptus 2 drops, Spanish sage 4 drops, Mandarin 4 drops

## Safety information

Eucalyptus is not recommended for people with epilepsy or allergy-prone skin.

# manuka *Leptospermum scoparium*

Manuka essential oil has an unusual aroma, warm and spicy with sharp, slightly medicinal but fresh undertones as it evaporates. It is soothing to the spirit, opening the airways to encourage slow, calm breaths.

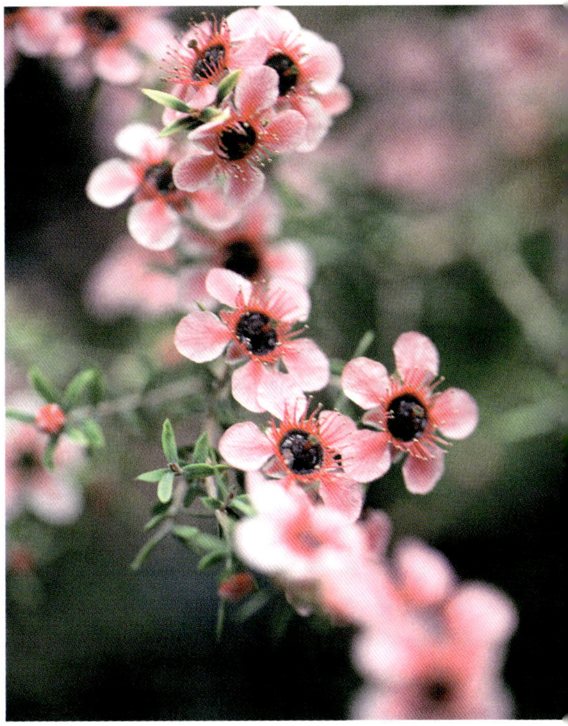

### Botanical source and background

A member of the Myrtaceae family, which includes many aromatic trees and shrubs, the manuka is a vigorous tree with highly aromatic, narrow-bladed green leaves, and is found only in New Zealand. Manuka is not commercially cultivated, so all available essential oil is produced by harvesting leaves and twigs from wild-growing trees. It replenishes itself easily so it is a sustainable source. The Maoris of New Zealand have used manuka leaves for centuries to help heal damaged skin, wounds and skin ulcers. They drink manuka tea as a remedy for head colds and to reduce fever, and rub a poultice made from manuka leaves and bark on aching joints. Honey made from manuka blossoms is useful in wound-healing, and helps to boost immunity to viral infections. Manuka is related to Australian tea tree; the two oils share similar properties and uses.

### Extraction and storage

Steam distillation of the leaves and twigs yields a pale yellow essential oil, which will last up to two years in the refrigerator, and one year at cool room temperature (54°F/12°C).

### Physical and psychological effects

*Antiseptic:* heals cuts, insect bites, acne, and fungal infections such as athlete's foot
*Immune-boosting:* builds resistance to fight viral infections such as flu
*Analgesic:* eases muscular aches and pains, stiffness or backache
*Expectorant:* helps tight, sore or mucousy coughs
*Nervous restorative:* eases depleted and stressed nerves

### Special manuka blends, in 4tsp (20ml) carrier oil

*Damaged-skin repair:* Manuka 4 drops, Myrrh 2 drops, Lavender 4 drops
*Immune tonic:* Manuka 4 drops, Ginger 2 drops, Lemon 4 drops
*Muscle-reliever:* Manuka 4 drops, Cardamom 4 drops, Black pepper 2 drops
*Chest-soother:* Manuka 4 drops, Eucalyptus 2 drops, Atlas cedarwood 4 drops
*Mental-revitalizer:* Manuka 4 drops, Mandarin 4 drops, Basil 2 drops

### Safety information

Manuka essential oil is non-toxic, non-irritating and non-sensitizing.

# tea tree *Melaleuca alternifolia*

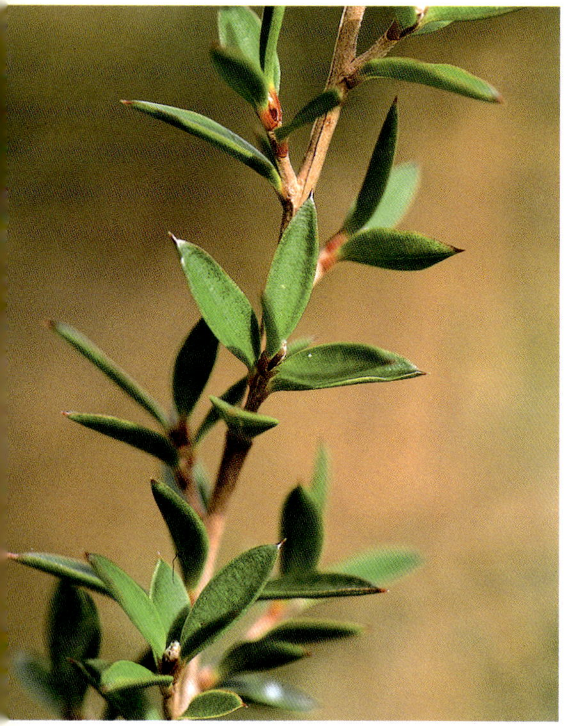

Tea tree essential oil has a strongly medicinal aroma which is also green, fresh and penetrating, with warmer and more herbal undertones as it evaporates. It is a very cleansing fragrance.

## Botanical source and background

Tea tree belongs to the Myrtaceae family, which includes many aromatic trees and shrubs. Native to Australia, it is a small tree or shrub, growing to 18ft (6m), with narrow aromatic leaves and yellowish-purple flowers. Unrelated to the tea plant from China or India popularly and drunk as a hot infusion (*Camellia sinensis*), tea tree is said to have acquired its common name in the 18th century when Captain Cook's crew drank an infusion of the leaves of *Melaleuca alternifolia* to prevent scurvy. Aboriginal Australians have used the leaves for centuries for colds, fevers and headaches. Commercial production of tea tree oil began in the early 20th century. It was regarded from the start as a highly efficient antiseptic, antimicrobial and antiviral agent with skin cleansing and disinfecting abilities.

## Extraction and storage

Steam distillation of the leaves and twigs yields a very pale yellow essential oil. Tea tree oil degrades quickly: it should be kept in the refrigerator where it will last up to one year. If kept at cool room temperature (54°F/12°C), it will last for six months.

## Physical and psychological effects

*Antimicrobial:* fights throat infections and fungal conditions such as athlete's foot
*Immune-boosting:* fights viral infections such as flu
*Expectorant:* clears chest congestion, eases coughs
*Wound-healer:* heals cracked or damaged skin
*Skin disinfectant:* heals infections such as acne and boils

## Special tea tree blends, in 4tsp (20ml) carrier oil

*Immune tonic:* Tea tree 4 drops, Lemon 4 drops, Myrtle 2 drops
*Chest relief:* Tea tree 4 drops, Black pepper 4 drops, Atlas cedarwood 2 drops
*Wound-healer:* Tea tree 4 drops, German chamomile 2 drops, Myrrh 4 drops
*Acne treatment:* Tea tree 4 drops, Frankincense 4 drops, Patchouli 2 drops

## Safety information

Some people have reported the occasional case of allergic skin reaction to tea tree, so use half the stated drops in the same amount of carrier oil on sensitive skin.

# peppermint *Mentha x piperita*

Peppermint essential oil has an extremely spicy, minty and fresh aroma with a penetrating menthol note, then warmer and sweeter undertones as it evaporates. It is a pungent and mouth-watering fragrance.

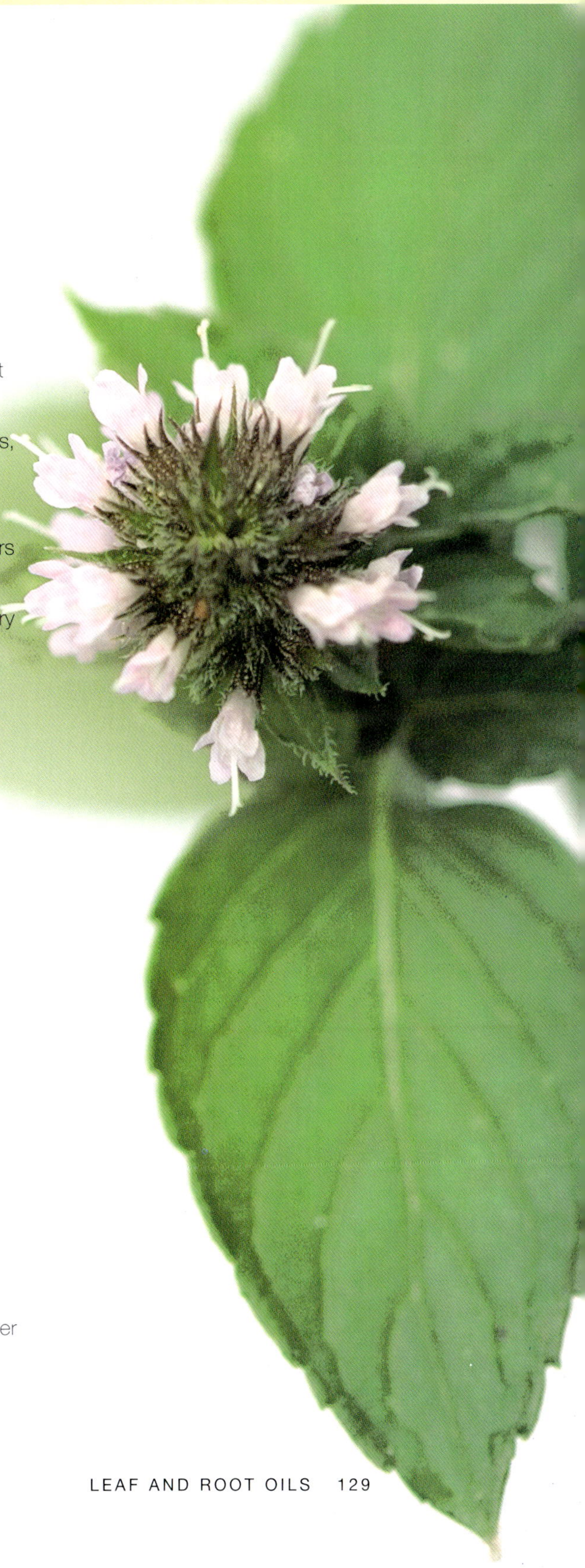

### Botanical source and background

Another member of the extensive Labiatae (Lamiaceae) family of aromatic herbs, peppermint is native to southern Europe and was introduced to North America in the 19th century. Cultivated on a commercial scale in France, Germany, Italy and Bulgaria, it is a hybrid cross between two species, probably spearmint (*Mentha spicata*) and water mint (*Mentha aquatica*). A vigorous herb up to 3ft (1m) in height, it has tough square stems, aromatic dark green leaves and tall spikes of purplish flowers. The Romans liked mint; they used it in sauces, wove it into garlands and wore it at feasts. Culpeper said in his famous 17th-century *Complete Herbal* "All the mints are astringent and great strengtheners of the stomach." The district of Mitcham in Surrey, England, was noted in the 18th and 19th centuries as one of the finest peppermint-producing areas in the world. This industry has now declined completely and the US is the largest global producer of the oil.

### Extraction and storage

Steam distillation of the leaves yields a very pale essential oil, which will last up to two years in the refrigerator and up to one year at cool room temperature (54°F/12°C).

### Physical and psychological effects

*Analgesic:* eases aches, muscle spasms or strains, or backache
*Antispasmodic:* soothes stomach cramps and indigestion
*Digestive tonic:* increases secretion of digestive juices; helps nausea or travel sickness
*Mentally-refreshing:* refreshes the mind, wakes up the senses

### Special peppermint blends, in 4tsp (20ml) carrier oil

*Muscle-reliever:* Peppermint 2 drops, Spanish sage 4 drops, Lavender 4 drops
*Stomach-soother:* Peppermint 2 drops, Ginger 4 drops, Coriander seed 4 drops
*Mental-rejuvenator:* Peppermint 2 drops, Rosemary 4 drops, May chang 4 drops

### Safety information

Peppermint oil is generally non-toxic, non-irritating and non-sensitizing. However, it is a powerful oil and best avoided in facial massage because it tends to make the eyes water profusely, and it is too strong for delicate skin.

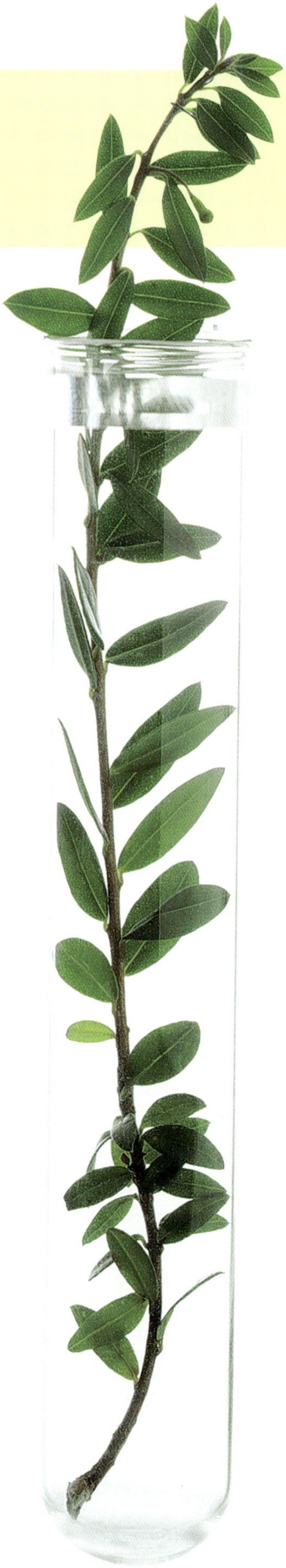

# myrtle *Myrtus communis*

Myrtle essential oil has a sharp, green and fresh aroma with bright citrus-like notes, becoming sweeter and lighter on evaporation. Sunny and fresh, it instantly lifts the spirit and cheers the mind.

## Botanical source and background

Myrtle is a member of the Myrtaceae family of aromatic trees and shrubs. It is native to the southern Mediterranean and is grown commercially for essential-oil production in France, Tunisia, Spain, Morocco and Corsica. A vigorous bush up to 3ft (1m) tall with reddish bark and stems, it has highly aromatic, small, lance-shaped, shiny, dark green leaves. It also produces small white flowers and black berries. In Ancient Greece, myrtle was linked to Aphrodite, the goddess of love and beauty, and burned as incense on her altars. To this day, sprigs of the plant are carried in wedding bouquets as an aromatic symbol of love. Myrtle has long been a traditional remedy for Mediterranean women, drunk as a tea to help tone the menstrual cycle, and used to make skin balms. Inhalations of myrtle leaves boiled in water are also used as an expectorant to help coughs and colds.

## Extraction and storage

Steam distillation of yarrow leaves and twigs yields a pale yellow or greenish essential oil, which will keep for up to two years in the refrigerator, and up to one year at cool room temperature (54°F/12°C).

## Physical and psychological effects

*Skin tonic:* astringent and toning, particularly for oily, combination or mature skins
*Expectorant:* soothes dry, sore or tickly coughs
*Immune-boosting:* strengthens resistance to colds and flu
*Antidepressant:* eases anxiety and nervous tension

## Special myrtle blends, in 4tsp (20ml) carrier oil

*Oily/combination facial treat:* Myrtle 2 drops, Geranium 2 drops, Neroli 1 drop
*Mature facial treat:* Myrtle 2 drops, Rose absolute 1 drop, Frankincense 2 drops
*Chest-soother:* Myrtle 4 drops, Atlas cedarwood 4 drops, Myrrh 2 drops
*Immune tonic:* Myrtle 4 drops, Manuka 4 drops, Ginger 2 drops
*Mood-enhancer:* Myrtle 4 drops, Mandarin 4 drops, Rose otto 2 drops

## Safety information

Myrtle essential oil is non-toxic, non-irritating and non-sensitizing.

# basil *Ocimum basilicum*

Basil essential oil has a penetrating, green and spicy aroma, with a warm note similar to clove. It becomes sweeter and softer as it evaporates. The oil has a mouth-watering freshness and tempts the appetite.

### Botanical source and background

Basil belongs to the Labiatae (Lamiaceae) family which includes all the Mediterranean herbs. It is native to the Far East and many species are found in different countries. *Ocimum basilicum* is the European basil, sometimes called "sweet basil", which is grown commercially in France, Italy and Eastern Europe as a culinary herb and for the essential oil. A vigorous annual, up to 2ft (60cm) in height, it has four-sided stems, and oval-shaped leaves that become more aromatic in hot temperatures and bright sunlight. Basil produces tall spikes of white flowers toward the end of summer. The Indian species *Ocimum sanctum* (Holy basil) has been regarded as sacred to the god Vishnu for centuries and many families grow it in their gardens for luck. In early western European herbal medicine basil was used as an remedy for poisonous bites from snakes, bees or wasps. Today, it is best known as a fragrant ingredient in Mediterranean cookery.

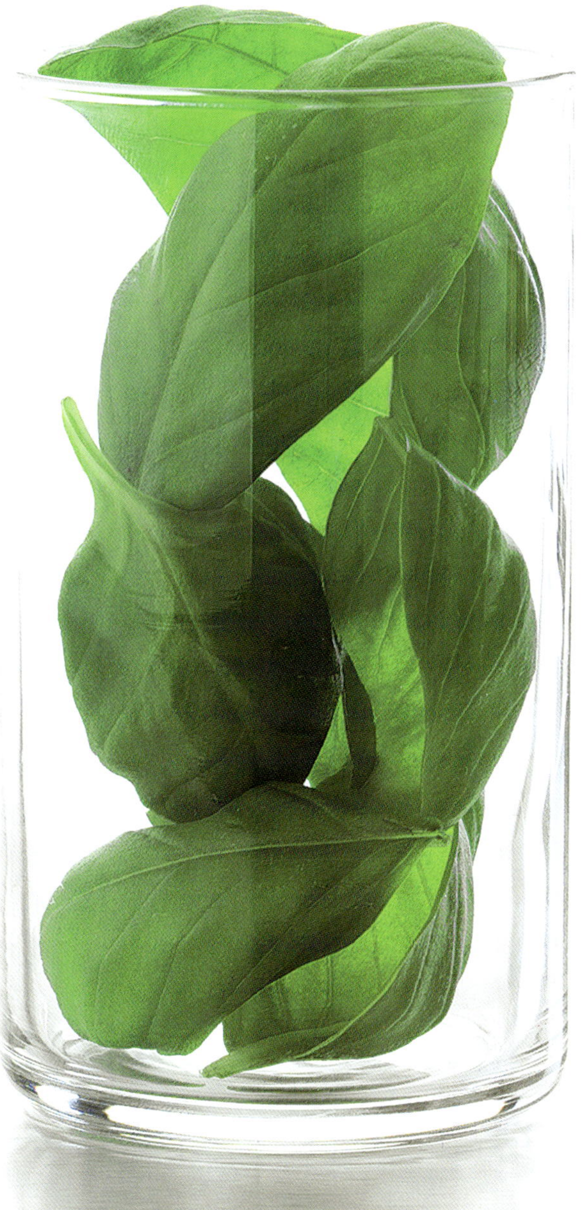

### Extraction and storage

Steam distillation of the leaves and stalks yields a colourless essential oil, which lasts for up to two years in the refrigerator, or one year at cool room temperature (54°F/12°C).

### Physical and psychological effects

*Digestive tonic:* eases indigestion, stomach aches and constipation
*Insect repellent:* repels mosquitoes and soothes itching bites
*Immune-boosting:* soothes chest infections, colds and flu
*Mentally-reviving:* rejuvenates and stimulates the mind

### Special basil blends, in 4tsp (20ml) carrier oil

*Digestive-soother:* Basil 2 drops, Sweet orange 6 drops, Ginger 2 drops
*Insect repellent:* Basil 2 drops, Lavender 4 drops, May chang 4 drops
*Immune tonic:* Basil 2 drops, Manuka 4 drops, Myrtle 4 drops
*Mental-refresher:* Basil 2 drops, Mandarin 4 drops, Petitgrain 4 drops

### Safety information

Basil essential oil should be avoided in pregnancy because it contains methyl charicol, a powerful chemical constituent which could pose a toxicity risk for the unborn child.

# sweet marjoram *Origanum marjorana*

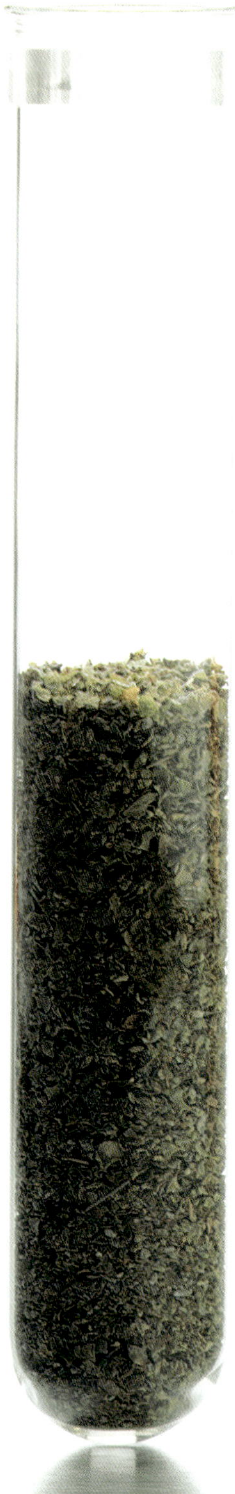

Sweet marjoram essential oil has a warm, herbal and sweet aroma with woody, nutty and spicy undertones. It is a pleasant and long-lasting fragrance with soothing effects on the spirit.

## Botanical source and background

Sweet marjoram belongs to the Labiatae (Lamiaceae) family of Mediterranean herbs. This species is native to the southern Mediterranean, but its essential oil is produced mostly in Tunisia, Morocco, Egypt and parts of Eastern Europe. A bushy perennial herb up to 2ft (60cm) tall, it has velvety stems, small aromatic leaves and tiny whitish flowers. The whole plant gives off a warm, herbal scent. Sweet marjoram essential oil should not be confused with Spanish marjoram which is actually a type of thyme with totally different properties and uses. Marjoram has been a popular culinary and medicinal herb for centuries. Its botanical name comes from the Ancient Greek *oros ganos*, which means "joy of the mountain". Greek physicians used it as an antidote to poison. In 16th-century Europe, bags of "swete marjerome" were used to scent bathwater and wash the body. Culpeper, the 17th-century English herbalist, regarded it as a soothing herb for the mind.

## Extraction and storage

Steam distillation of the dried leaves and flowers yields a pale yellow essential oil. It lasts for up to two years in the refrigerator, and one year at cool room temperature (54°F/12°C).

## Physical and psychological effects

*Antispasmodic:* eases stomach cramps, menstrual pain, indigestion or constipation
*Analgesic:* helps headaches or muscular aches and pains
*Expectorant:* soothes irritated and sore coughs
*Calming:* soothes fraught and over-excited emotions; calms strong feelings such as grief

## Special marjoram blends, in 4tsp (20ml) carrier oil

*Abdominal-soother:* Sweet marjoram 4 drops, Lavender 4 drops, German chamomile 2 drops
*Pain-reliever:* Sweet marjoram 4 drops, Roman chamomile 4 drops, Peppermint 2 drops
*Chest massage:* Sweet marjoram 4 drops, Myrtle 4 drops, Cardamom 2 drops
*Emotional support:* Sweet marjoram 4 drops, Neroli 2 drops, Sandalwood 4 drops

## Safety information

Sweet marjoram oil is non-toxic, non-irritating and non-sensitizing.

# geranium *Pelargonium graveolens*

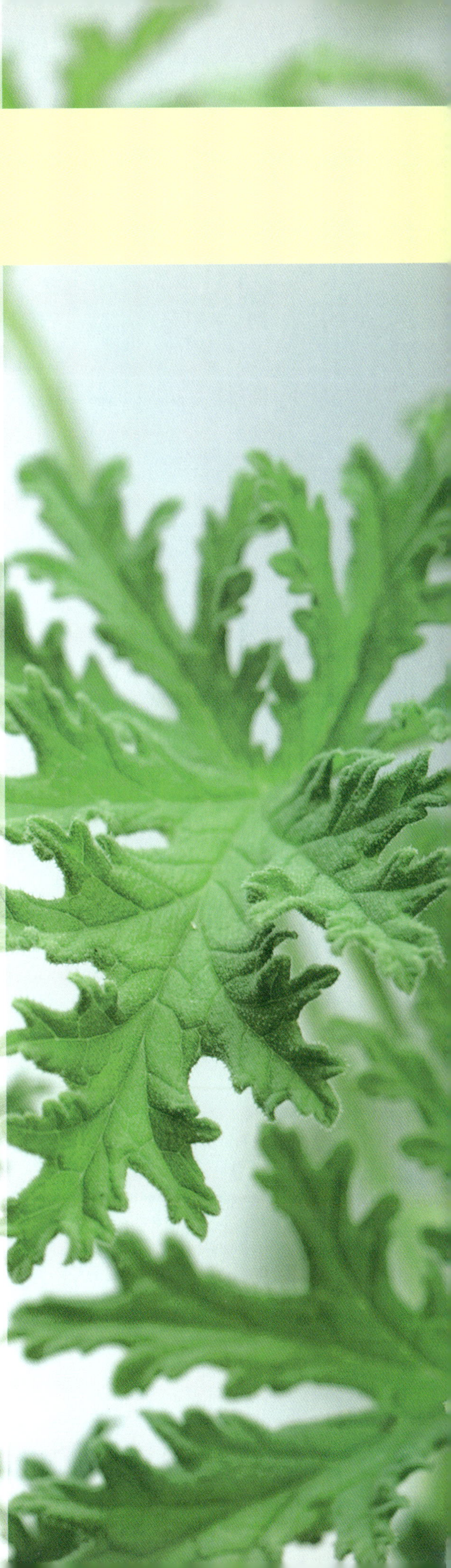

Geranium essential oil has a green, fresh and sweet aroma, with a strong rosy note, becoming very sweet as it evaporates. Light and soft, it soothes the spirit and eases mental stress.

### Botanical source and background

A member of the Geraniaceae family, this type of geranium is originally from South Africa. It was introduced to many countries and hybridized into many varieties in the 17th and 18th centuries. *Pelargonium graveolens* is a tropical plant with velvety, highly rose-scented leaves and tiny pinkish flowers. Today, the best-quality geranium oil is called "Bourbon Geranium" and comes from Réunion, Egypt and China. Geranium is a name which has been known since Ancient Greek times – it comes from the Greek for crane, a bird with a long beak. This was said to refer to the long seed pods produced by true geranium species. When pelargoniums were discovered in the 17th century in South Africa, rather confusingly they were also given the common name "geranium". *Pelargonium graveolens* and similar species have been used extensively in the perfumery industry since the 19th century because of their strong rosy aroma.

### Extraction and storage

Steam distillation of the fresh leaves yields a pale yellow essential oil, which will keep for up to two years in the refrigerator, and one year at cool room temperature (54°F/12°C).

### Physical and psychological efffects

*Skin-toning:* balances the production of the skin's oil making it an excellent tonic for dry, oily or mature skins
*Hormone-balancing:* balances the menstrual hormones, easing PMS symptoms such as fluid retention, breast tenderness and mood swings
*Skin-healing:* repairs damaged, very dry or thin skin
*Antidepressant:* uplifts negative feelings, easing mental or emotional stress

### Special geranium blends, in 4tsp (20ml) carrier oil

*Special facial treatment:* Geranium 2 drops, Rosewood 2 drops, Neroli 1 drop
*Hormone-balancer:* Geranium 4 drops, May chang 2 drops, Sandalwood 4 drops
*Skin repair:* Geranium 4 drops, Frankincense 4 drops, German chamomile 2 drops

### Safety information

Generally non-toxic and non-irritating, however, some cases of sensitization have been reported, so geranium essential oil is not advised for individuals with allergy-prone skin.

# scotch pine *Pinus sylvestris*

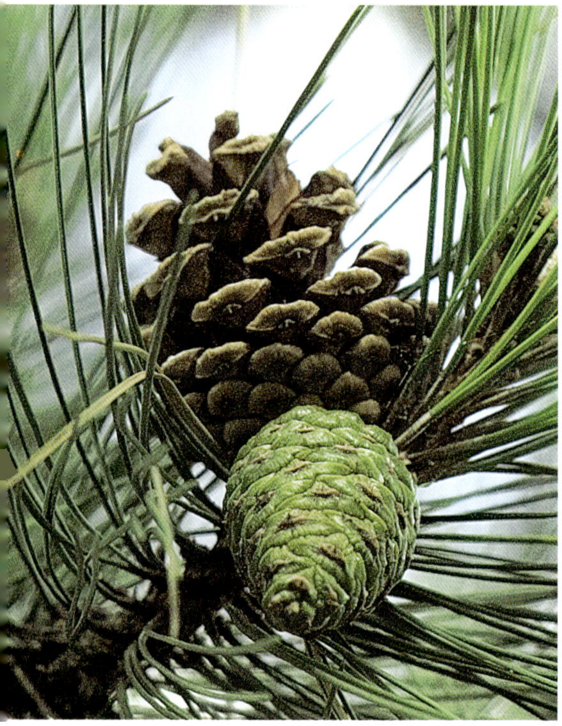

Scotch pine essential oil is a penetrating, green and fresh aroma with a strong medicinal undertone, becoming sweeter and woodier as it evaporates. It is a familiar fragrance with a very cleansing effect.

### Botanical source and background

A member of the Pinaceae family of evergreen trees, Scotch pine is grown in Russia, Finalnd, Austria, Germany and Hungary, where much of the essential oil is produced. It is an aromatic tree growing up to 120ft (40m), with reddish bark, a flat crown of branches, dark green needles and brown cones. The timber is used in construchtion and furniture-making, and the needles and twigs are used for essential-oil production. *Pinus sylvestris* provides the essential oil used in aromatherapy, but all other pine species are also aromatic and produce semi-solid resins, which have been used for centuries to help respiratory and sinus problems. In North America, indigenous peoples used the resin and twigs of local species as insect repellents and lice-proof bedding! Pine resins are also used in toiletry products.

### Extraction and storage

Steam distillation of the needles and twigs yields a colourless essential oil, which will last up to two years in the refrigerator, and up to one year at cool room temperature (54°F/12°C).

### Physical and psychological effects

*Circulatory stimulant:* warms cold hands and feet, and chilly limbs
*Analgesic:* helps aches and pains, muscular stiffness and rheumatic pain
*Respiratory tonic:* eases coughs and chest congestion
*Immune-boosting:* improves resistance to viral and bacterial infections
*Mentally-clearing:* clears the head; improves concentration

### Special Scotch pine blends, in 4tsp (20ml) carrier oil

*Circulation stimulant:* Scotch pine 2 drops, Black pepper 4 drops, May chang 4 drops
*Muscle-reliever:* Scotch pine 2 drops, Ginger 4 drops, Lavendin 4 drops
*Chest-soother:* Scotch pine 2 drops, Myrtle 4 drops, Atlas cedarwood 4 drops
*Immune tonic:* Scotch pine 2 drops, Lemon 4 drops, Spanish sage 4 drops
*Mental-rejuvenator:* Scotch pine 2 drops, Peppermint 2 drops, Grapefruit 6 drops

### Safety information

Scotch pine oil is regarded as non-toxic and non-irritant at stated doses; it is best avoided on individuals with highly allergy-prone skin.

# patchouli *Pogostemon cablin*

Patchouli essential oil has a woody and musky aroma, rich and sharp at first, with deeper, earthier and smoky undertones. A powerful and unusual fragrance, it is considered by many to be an aphrodisiac.

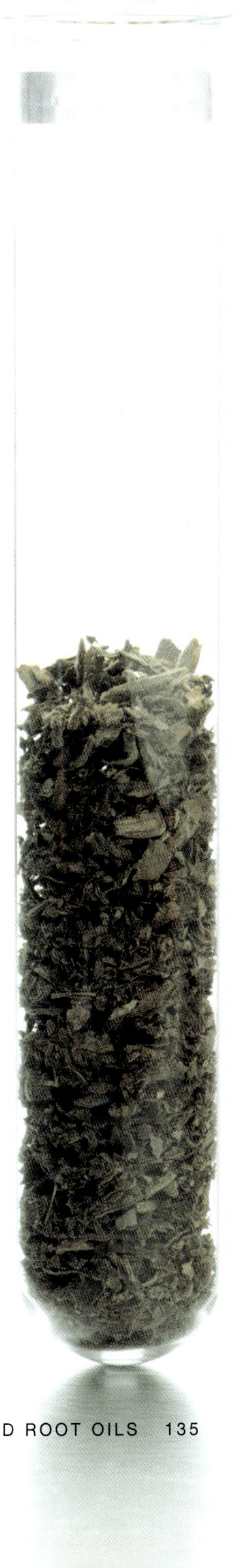

### Botanical source and background

Patchouli belongs to the Labiatae (Lamiaceae) plant family, and is native to tropical Asia, particularly Indonesia, which is a main producer of the oil. It is also grown commercially in India, the Philippines, Malaysia and China. A perennial herb up to 3ft (1m) tall, it has large, velvety, dark green leaves. Tiny hair-like projections on the leaf surface produce the essential oil, and rubbing them releases its fragrance. Patchouli has been used since ancient times in India, China and Japan as a perfume, incense and medicine. In traditional Eastern medicine, dried patchouli leaves are a remedy for colds, headaches and nausea. The herb has also been used for centuries to protect precious fabrics from moths. In India, patchouli oil and leaves are used in perfumes, cosmetics and incense. In the West, patchouli became popular in the 19th century when shawls scented with it were in fashion; it also gained fame in the 1960s when incense became part of popular culture.

### Extraction and storage

Steam distillation of the partially dried leaves yields a deep yellow, thick, sticky essential oil, which will last up to two years in the refrigerator, and up to one year at cool room temperature (54°F/12°C).

### Physical and psychological effects

*Skin-toning:* restores and deeply moisturizes dry, dull or mature skins
*Skin-healing:* heals deeply cracked, environmentally damaged skin or eczema
*Insect repellent:* helps repel mosquitoes
*Emotionally-stabilizing:* soothes emotional stress, eases fraught feelings

### Special patchouli blends, in 4tsp (20ml) carrier oil

*Special facial treatment:* Patchouli 1 drop, Rose absolute 1 drop, Frankincense 3 drops
*Skin repair:* Patchouli 2 drops, Myrrh 4 drops, Lavender 4 drops
*Insect repellent:* Patchouli 2 drops, Atlas cedarwood 4 drops, May chang 4 drops
*Emotional support:* Patchouli 2 drops, Jasmine 2 drops, Sweet orange 6 drops

### Safety information

Patchouli essential oil is non-toxic, non-irritating and non-sensitizing.

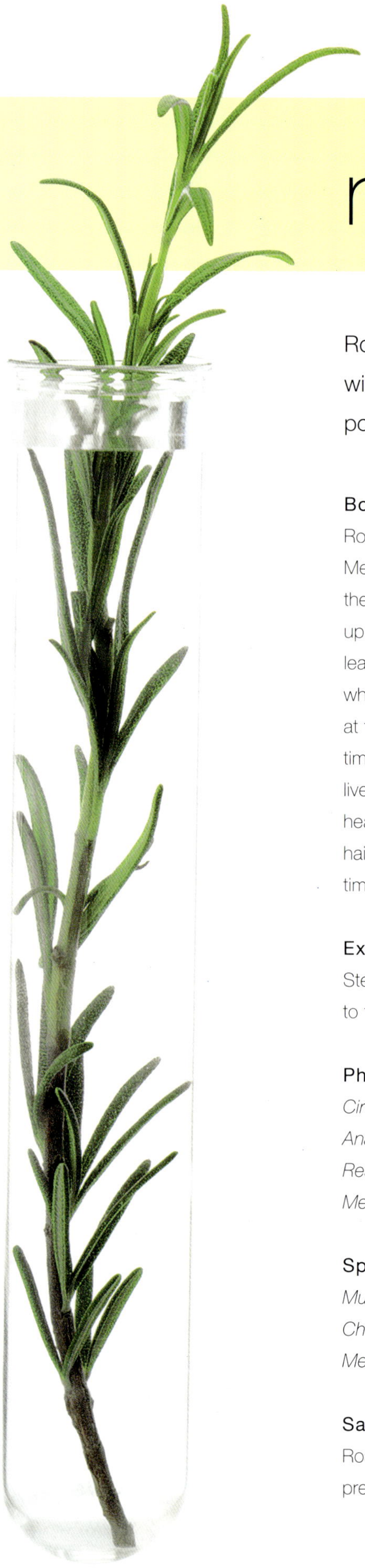

# rosemary *Rosmarinus officinalis*

Rosemary essential oil has a warm, herbal and camphoraceous aroma with woody and sweeter undertones as it evaporates. Pungent and powerful, it cuts through mental fog and improves concentration.

## Botanical source and background

Rosemary belongs to the large plant family Labiatae (Lamiaceae), which includes all the Mediterranean herbs. Native to the southern Mediterranean area, it is now grown all over the world. The essential oil is mainly produced in Spain, France and North Africa. Growing up to 6ft (2m), rosemary is a woody shrub that is highly aromatic because its slender green leaves are full of essential oil sacs. Different rosemary varieties produce blue, pale blue or white flowers in early spring. Rosemary is harvested at the height of summer when its oil is at the highest concentration. In Western Europe, rosemary has been used since ancient times as an incense and a medicinal remedy. Early Greek physicians recommended it for liver and digestive problems. In the 17th century, the English herbalist Culpeper used it for headaches, stomach pains, toothache and rheumatism. Rosemary is a traditional skin and hair tonic and is also an ingredient in the original eau-de-Cologne formula. In medieval times it was used in wedding bouquets, symbolizing fidelity between marriage partners.

## Extraction and storage

Steam distillation of rosemary leaves yields a colourless essential oil, which will keep for up to two years in the refrigerator, and one year at cool room temperature (54°F/12°C).

## Physical and psychological effects

*Circulatory tonic:* improves local circulation, and warms the skin and underlying muscles
*Analgesic*: eases backache, muscular spasms and pulls
*Respiratory tonic:* eases chest congestion, improves breathing and eases coughs
*Memory stimulant:* helps poor concentration, clears mental clutter

## Special rosemary blends, in 4tsp (20ml) carrier oil

*Muscle-reliever:* Rosemary 4 drops, Lemongrass 2 drops, Black pepper 4 drops
*Chest-comforter:* Rosemary 4 drops, Lemon 4 drops, Eucalyptus 2 drops
*Mental-awakener:* Rosemary 4 drops, Basil 2 drops, Peppermint 4 drops

## Safety information

Rosemary oil should not be used on pregnant women or people with epilepsy or high blood pressure. It has a stimulating effect on the mind and so is best used for daytime treatments.

# spanish sage *Salvia lavandulaefolia*

Spanish sage essential oil has a warm, sweet and pungent aroma with a unique blend of lavender and sage notes. It is woodier and softer on evaporation. Instantly fresh and reviving, the oil lifts the spirit.

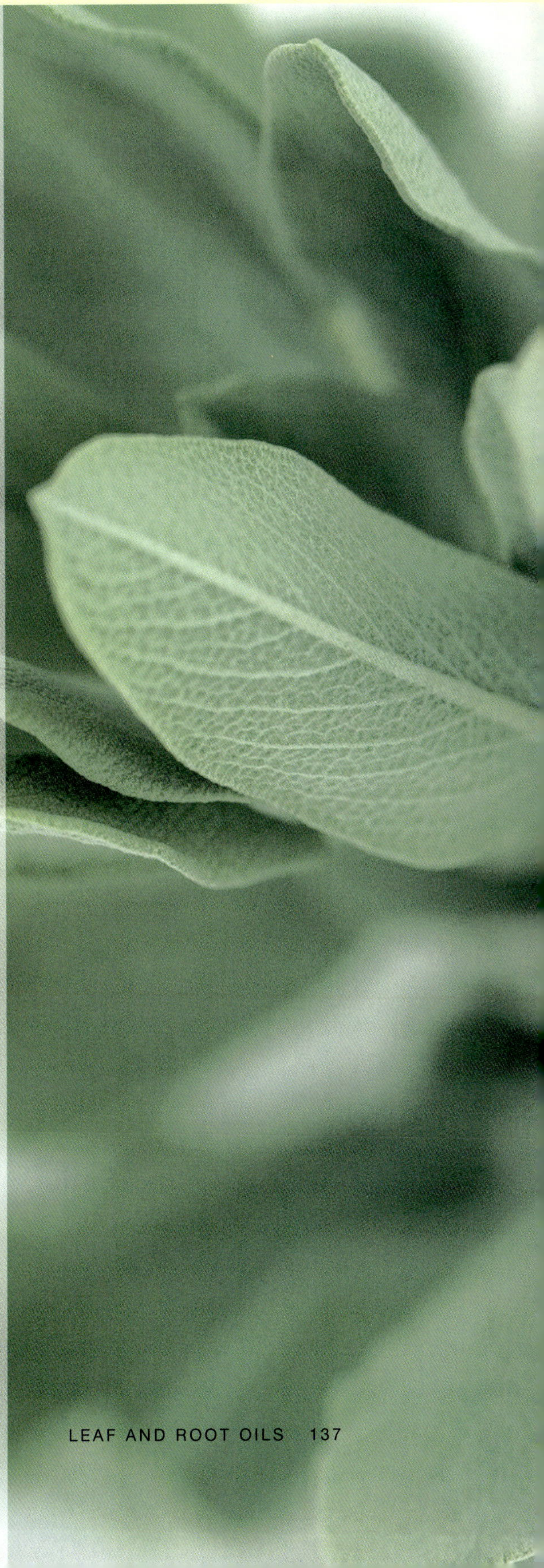

### Botanical source and background

Spanish sage belongs to the Labiatae (Lamiaceae) family of Mediterranean herbs, and is native to Spain, the only producer of the essential oil. It is a strong and vigorous perennial herb growing to 2ft (60cm), with soft, velvety, blueish-green leaves which are highly aromatic. The Latin name means "the sage with lavender-like leaves" because its aroma is a unique combination of lavender and sage. Spanish sage produces tall spikes of lilac-purple blooms in high summer, and it is more aromatic in hot, sunny conditions. It is mostly used in traditional herbal medicine as an anti-infectious remedy, helpful for all immune-related problems including chesty coughs and flu. Regarded as a powerful tonic to the system, it is also used to treat circulatory problems and rheumatic pain. Women use it to tone up the menstrual cycle and to relieve period pain or headaches.

### Extraction and storage

Steam distillation of the leaves yields a colourless essential oil. It will keep for up to two years in the refrigerator, and up to one year at cool room temperature (54°F/12°C).

### Physical and psychological effects

*Immune-boosting:* helps the body to resist bacterial and viral infections
*Expectorant:* eases breathing, clears congestion and soothes coughs
*Analgesic:* eases muscular aches and pains, and backache and rheumatic pains
*Menstrual tonic:* helps to regulate the menstrual cycle and eases period pain
*Antidepressant:* uplifts the mind and the emotions

### Special Spanish sage blends, in 4tsp (20ml) carrier oil

*Immune tonic:* Spanish sage 2 drops, Cardamom 4 drops, Nutmeg 4 drops
*Chest-reliever:* Spanish sage 2 drops, Atlas cedarwood 4 drops, Myrrh 4 drops
*Muscle-warmer:* Spanish sage 2 drops, Rosemary 4 drops, May chang 4 drops
*Menstrual-balancer:* Spanish sage 2 drops, Clary sage 4 drops, Mandarin 4 drops
*Antidepressant:* Spanish sage 2 drops, Lemon 4 drops, Frankincense 4 drops

### Safety information

Spanish sage is not to be used in pregnancy as it stimulates the muscles of the uterus.

# vetiver *Vetiveria zizanoides*

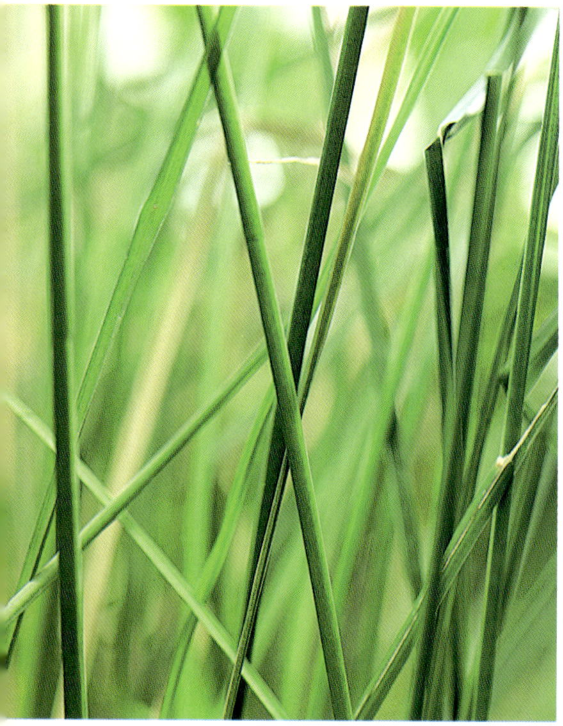

Vetiver has a most unusual aroma – very deep, smoky and earthy, and persistent and powerful, with slightly richer, sweeter undertones. Its exotic depth lingers on the skin.

## Botanical source and background

A member of the vast Gramineae plant family, vetiver is native to Indonesia, India and Sri Lanka. It is now also grown in South America, the Philippines and Réunion. It is a tropical grass up to 3ft (1m) tall, with sharp-edged blades and a large interlaced root system. In India it is cultivated to help stop soil erosion as well as for its roots, which yield the essential oil. The aroma of vetiver helps to repel moths, so the oil is used to scent cloth or carpets, often in combination with patchouli. It is also used as an ingredient in many powdered incense combinations, especially in India and Sri Lanka. In the West, vetiver is best known as a fragrance compound, in great demand for men's toiletries and, as a "fixative", or strong heavy note, in oriental or exotic perfume formulae.

## Extraction and storage

Steam distillation of the roots yields a very dark brown, sticky and thick essential oil, which will keep for up to two years in the refrigerator, and up to one year at cool room temperature (54°F/12°C).

## Physical and psychological effects

*Muscle relaxant:* eases muscle spasm, severe aches and pains and backache
*Mild circulatory tonic:* improves circulation and eases physical stiffness
*Reproductive tonic:* eases pre-menstrual symptoms such as mood swings, depression and lethargy; in menopausal women it helps tiredness and fluctuating energy levels
*Skin-toning:* tones and restores tired, slack skin and balances excess oil production
*Grounding and stabilizing:* soothes and calms deep anxiety or emotional tension

## Special vetiver blends, in 4tsp (20ml) carrier oil

*Muscle-relaxer:* Vetiver 2 drops, Lavender 4 drops, Ginger 4 drops
*Hormone-balancer:* Vetiver 2 drops, Geranium 4 drops, Mandarin 4 drops
*Mature skin treatment:* Vetiver 1 drop, Rose absolute 1 drop, Sandalwood 3 drops
*Emotional soother:* Vetiver 2 drops, Rosewood 4 drops, Atlas cedarwood 4 drops

## Safety information

Vetiver essential oil is non-toxic, non-irritating and non-sensitizing.

# ginger *Zingiber officinale*

Ginger essential oil has a sweet, sharp and soft aroma, with rich and spicy undertones. It smells much sweeter than fresh ginger root, and its pungency develops as the fragrance evaporates on the skin.

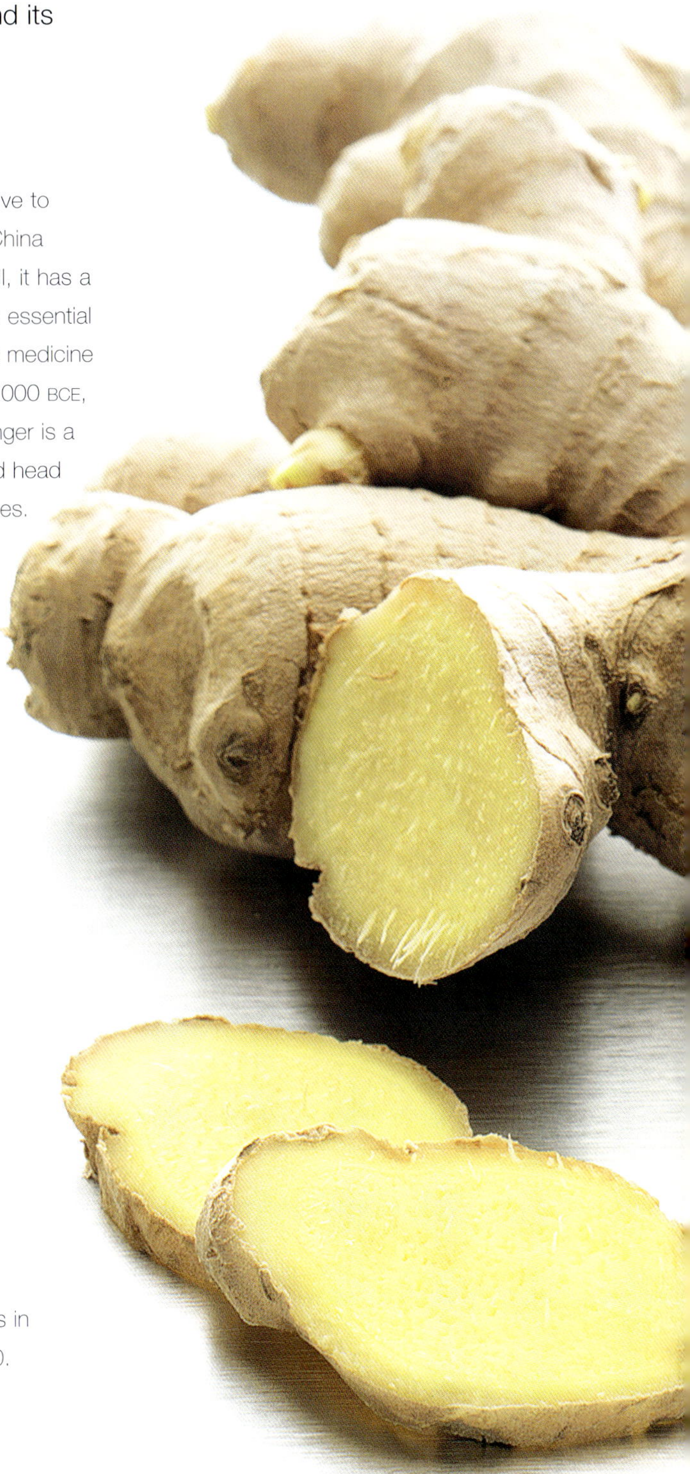

### Botanical source and background

A member of the Zingiberaceae family, which includes many spices, ginger is native to Southeast Asia. Today, it is cultivated in the West Indies, as well as in India and China where the essential oil is produced. An attractive tropical plant up to 5ft (1.5m) tall, it has a graceful erect stem, pairs of lance-shaped leaves and aromatic white flowers. The essential oil is found in the fleshy root. In the Far East, ginger has been used in cookery and medicine for thousands of years. It is mentioned in a Chinese medical text dating back to 2000 BCE, and was a staple remedy and flavouring in ancient India. In Ayurvedic medicine ginger is a hot and dry cure, rebalancing cold and moist conditions such as runny noses and head colds. Ginger was used in medieval Europe to flavour both sweet and savoury dishes.

### Extraction and storage

Steam distillation of the dried root yields a virtually colourless essential oil. It lasts up to two years in the refrigerator, and one year at cool room temperature (54°F/12°C).

### Physical and psychological effects

*Digestive tonic:* eases stomach cramps, indigestion and constipation
*Immune-boosting:* builds resistance to viral or bacterial infections
*Expectorant:* eases tight, sore or mucousy coughs
*Circulatory stimulant:* warms cold hands and feet or chilly limbs
*Emotionally-warming:* soothes negative feelings, releases emotional tension

### Special ginger blends, in 4tsp (20ml) carrier oil

*Digestive-soother:* Ginger 2 drops, Cardamom 4 drops, Mandarin 4 drops
*Immune tonic:* Ginger 2 drops, Manuka 4 drops, Lemon 4 drops
*Chest relief:* Ginger 2 drops, Atlas cedarwood 4 drops, Myrrh 4 drops
*Emotional soother:* Ginger 2 drops, Neroli 2 drops, Sweet orange 6 drops

### Safety information

Ginger is non toxic and non-irritant at low doses; do not exceed the stated drops in blends. Avoided using on highly allergy-prone skin and also on children under 10.

# useful addresses

**Aromatherapy associations:**
Contact these associations to find a recognized practitioner or information about professional training courses.

**In the UK**

*British Complementary Medicine Association (BCMA)*
PO Box 5122, Bournemouth BH8 0WG
Tel: (0845) 345 5977
www.bcma.co.uk

*International Federation of Professional Aromatherapists (IFPA)*
82 Ashby Road, Hinckley
Leicestershire LE10 1SN
Tel: (01455) 637987
www.ifparoma.org

*International Therapy Examination Council (ITEC)*
4 Heathfield Terrace
London W4 4JE
Tel: (020) 8994 4141
www.itecworld.co.uk

**In the USA**

*IMA Group (International Massage Association Inc.)*
PO Box 421, 25 South Fourth Street
Warrenton VA 20188-0421
Tel: (540) 351 0800
www.imagroup.com

*American Massage Therapy Association (AMTA)*
500 Davis St, Suite 900,
Evanston IL 60201-4695
Tel: (847) 864 0123
www.amtamassage.org

*National Association for Holistic Aromatherapy*
4509 Interlake Ave N. #233
Seattle, WA 98103-6773
Tel: (206) 547 2164
www.naha.org

**In the Canada**

*Canadian Federation of Aromatherapists (CFA)*
1136 Centre Street, Suite 207
Thornhill, Ontario L4J 7M8
Tel: (905) 886 2567 (519) 746-1594
www.cfacanada.com

**In the Australia**

*International Federation of Aromatherapists. Australian Branch*
PO Box 786, Templestowe, VIC 3106
Tel (61) 3 9850 9524
www.ifa.org.au

**Essential oil suppliers**

*Aromatherapy Products Ltd*
Newtown Road, Hove BN3 7BA, UK
Tel: (01273) 325666
www.tisserand.com

*Essentially Oils Ltd*
8–10 Mount Farm, Junction Rd
Churchill, Oxfordshire OX7 6NP, UK
Tel: (01608) 659544
www.essentiallyoils.com

# further reading

Harding, Jennie, *Secrets of Aromatherapy*, Dorling Kindersley, London, (UK), 2000

Tisserand, Robert, *The Art of Aromatherapy*, CW Daniels, Saffron Walden, Essex (UK), 1977

Lawless, Julia, *The Illustrated Encyclopedia of Essential Oils*, Element Books, Shaftesbury, Dorset (UK) 1995

Rose, Jeanne, *375 Essential oils and Hydrosols*, Frog, Berkeley, CA (US), 1999

Davis, Patricia, *A-Z of Aromatherapy*, CW Daniels, Saffron Walden, Essex (UK), 1995

George, Mike, *Learn to Relax*, Duncan Baird Publishers, London (UK) and Chronicle, San Francisco, CA (US) 1998

Smith, Karen, *Massage*, Duncan Baird Publishers, London (UK), 1998 and Thorsons, New York (US) 2002

# index

Page numbers for the main descriptions of oils are given in **bold**

# acknowledgments

**AUTHOR'S ACKNOWLEDGMENTS**

I would like to thank Robert Tisserand for being my original guide, teacher and inspiration in aromatherapy; also my colleagues, friends and students at the Tisserand Institute for all the years of learning and growing together.

**PICTURE ACKNOWLEDGMENTS**

The publisher would like to thank the following people, museums and photographic libraries for permission to reproduce their material. Every care has been taken to trace copyright holders. However, if we have omitted anyone we apologize and will, if informed, make corrections to any future edition.

**Page 17** Julie Toy/Getty Images; **20** S. Pitamitz/Zefa; **26** David Raymer/Corbis; **39** Pinto/Zefa; **48** D. Tardif/LWA/Zefa; **51** Alan Veldenzer/Photolibrary.com; **51** Neovision/Photonica; **90** Deni Bown/OSF/Photolibrary.com; **105** Garden World Images, Essex; **113** Edward Parker, Dorset; **127** Kelly Kalhoefer/OSF/Photolibrary.com; **128** Dave Watts/NHPA, Sussex.

**PUBLISHER'S ACKNOWLEDGMENTS**

The publishers would also like to thank the following people and organizations for their help in the production of this book:

G. Baldwin & Co.

The Tisserand Institute

The Royal Botanic Gardens, Kew

Models: Jasmine Hemsley, Amanda Wright (hands)

Make-up artist: Tinks Reding

Stylist: Vida Smallwood